Herbal Combinations

The Natural Harmony of Combining Herbs

by Rita Elkins, M.A.

Woodland Publishing
Pleasant Grove, UT

Woodland Publishing
P.O. Box 160
Pleasant Grove, UT
84062

CONTENTS

Introduction   5

The Nervous System   7
(Herbal Formula One)

The Gastro-Intestinal System   .   .   .   14
(Herbal Formula Two)

Colon Cleanser   19
(Herbal Formula Three)

Systemic Cleanser for Internal Organs   .   27
(Herbal Formula Four)

The Cardiovascular System   .   .   .   32
(Herbal Formula Five)

The Respiratory System   34
(Herbal Formula Six)

The Respiratory and Gastro-Intestinal Systems   38
(Herbal Formula Seven)

The Urinary System   42
(Herbal Formula Eight)

The Female Reproductive System . . 47
(Herbal Formula Nine)

Tonic and Energizing Herbs for all Systems . 56
(Herbal Formula Ten)

Endnotes 59

HERBAL COMBINATIONS

The Natural Harmony of Combining Herbs

TEN OF THE MOST EFFECTIVE HERBAL COMBINATIONS

Introduction

For centuries Chinese herbalists understood that prescribing herbs in time-tested formulas was much more effective than using single botanical preparations. The widespread use of various herbal formulations resulted in the compilation of several thousand herbal blends. Traditionally, these blends were individually adjusted according to the needs of the patient. The time-honored practice of carefully designing herbal formulations is based on the concept of synergistic enhancement. In other words, certain plants exist in nature which function more efficiently when they merge their medicinal attributes.

The Beauty of Herbal Blending

Today, scientific research supports the ancient idea of herbal "marriages." The notion that combining certain herbs together creates a better therapeutic effect can be supported by clinical studies. It's important to remember that the interaction between certain botanicals can be even more important than the individual properties of each contributing herb. Well-designed herbal formulas can exert impressive therapeutic effects on a number of maladies. These actions can be quite dramatic and don't have the negative side effects of synthetic pharmaceutical preparations.

Herbal Formulas: Balancing the Yin and the Yang

Herbal formulas can include from just two herbs to as many as twenty. The reasoning behind combining specific herbs together is based on the need to potentiate and balance the therapeutic action of each herb. Frequently, single herbs may be quite strong and require a form of buffering or balancing. Adding demulcent or carminative herbs improves the digestibility of other herbs, thereby enhancing their systemic action. Frequently, a single herb does not always possess certain properties needed to address specific symptoms. Consequently, other selected herbs are added, thereby creating a complete formula designed to precisely target certain body systems. One of the advantages of blending herbs is that various symptoms can be treated simultaneously.

Most herbal blends are comprised of what might be called dominant, more active plants, which are usually responsible for primary therapeutic actions, combined with more passive herbs that serve to soothe, support and potentiate. Stimulatory herbs are usually of the bitter variety and are very nicely complemented by aromatic, carminative and demulcent herbs. For example; Senna is a stimulatory and dynamic bitter herb which initiates colon muscle contraction. Adding Ginger, a carminative, to Senna serves to soothe the stomach and prevent gripping which may occur if Senna was taken alone. The addition of Capsicum or Ginger to any herb formula acts as a catalyst, increasing the efficiency of each individual herb. Herbs like Peppermint are potentiated by Capsicum. Moreover, the menthol contained in Peppermint helps to balance out the "hot" nature of the Capsicum. A good herbal blend will combine stimulant herbs with nourishing, protecting and cleansing varieties.

How Herbal Combinations Are Designed

The best herbal blends are based on the idea of synergy and balance and must be carefully formulated for optimal results. Judiciously assessing the nature of each herb is essential. For example; herbs have a number of different actions or characters. Herbs can be antispasmodic, analgesic, antibiotic, diuretic, emetic, cathartic, laxative, stimulant, tonic etc. Assessing the symptoms and body systems affected by disease or injury is necessary to create the appropriate mix of various herbs.

In order to gain the maximum effect from certain types of herbs, their chemical constituents must be combined. In so doing, they are potentiated and balanced, creating an herbal formulation that takes advantages of Mother Nature's natural pharmaceutical agents. The following sections will be divided according to body systems with recommended herbal combinations which have been designed to target specific physiological functions.

Advantages of Herbal Blending

• Combined herbs will have more than one function
• The physiological effects of combined herbs can treat disorders without the side effects of pharmaceutical drugs
• The biochemical reactions triggered by herbal blends can continue to enhance health even after the combination is no longer taken.
•Herbal combinations target the root of the disease rather than mask its symptoms.
• Herbs are naturally derived compounds that chemically complement each other by balancing and potentiating.
• The addition of other nutrients to herbal blends can also help to accelerate their therapeutic effect.

THE NERVOUS SYSTEM

DISORDERS TARGETED: insomnia, anxiety, nervous tension, stress, pain, muscle cramping, sleep disorders, hyperexcitability, psychosomatic disturbances, back spasms, headaches, panic attacks

Herbal Formula One

Hops, Valerian Root, Chamomile, Skullcap, Black Cohosh, Marshmallow, Wood Betony and Mullein

This formula combines the best nervine herbs available in a blend of sedative, anti-spasmodic and tonic herbs to create a calming effect on the nervous system. While each of these herbs is valuable individually, taking them alone is less effective. When mixed, they each contribute individual actions which serve to enhance and strengthen their combined effect. Insomnia and restlessness frequently result from stress, muscle cramping, stomach upset, pain or anxiety. The use of prescription hypnotics and tranquilizers pose a substantial risk and are often highly addictive. Nature provides excellent natural, sedative alternatives which promote satisfying rest and relaxation without a whole host of deleterious side effects.

Combing herbs that target symptoms associated with insomnia or anxiety creates the optimal therapeutic blend. In this case:

• Hops works to alleviate restless and pain.
• Valerian contributes superb natural sedative actions.
• Skullcap inhibits muscle spasms and cramping.
• Black Cohosh quiets irritable nerves.
• Marshmallow plays a supporting protective role by soothing and quieting the gastrointestinal tract.
• Wood Betony relaxes and dilates blood vessels.
• Chamomile eases anxiety by augmenting the tranquilizing effects of this formula with its carminative action.

Individual Herbs

HOPS (HUMULUS LUPULUS)

OVERVIEW: Used for centuries by herbalists, Native Americans prescribed the blossom for its sedative effect and dried it for relieving the pain of toothaches. Ancient Romans relied on Hops to promote sleep and relieve restlessness. Today, the medicinal use of Hops for sleep promotion is well documented.
CHARACTER: nervine, sedative, stomachic, carminative and cholagogue
ACTIVE COMPOUNDS: Lupulin, a chemical compound is found in the flower cones of Hops. Volatile oils, (humulene, myrcene, B-carophyllene, and farnescene), flavnonoids (rutin, quercitin and astragalin), resins (2-Methyl-3 butonol, humulone, lumulone, lupulone and vaeronic acid), and bitter acids are also contained in the herb.
MEDICINAL APPLICATIONS: insomnia, anxiety, nervousness, pain, stress, stomach spasms, inflammation, and colon disorders
SCIENTIFIC UPDATES: Recent in-depth clinical studies have revealed that Hops works to relax smooth muscle and naturally sedates the nervous system. Lupulone and humulone are the active ingredients of Hops responsible for its sedative properties.[1, 2,3,4] The flavonoid content gives Hops its anti-inflammatory action.
SAFETY: Hops has no known toxicity. It is not recommended for anyone who is suffering from clinical depression.
COMPLEMENTARY AGENTS: Valerian Root, Skullcap, Chamomile, Mullein, Marshmallow, Wood Betony, Passion Flower, Vitamin E, B-complex, Folic Acid, Niacin, Vitamin C, inositol, Calcium/ Magnesium, and Melatonin

VALERIAN ROOT (VALERIANA OFFICINALIS)

OVERVIEW: Valerian Root has been used since the time of the ancient Greeks as a sleep aid and antispasmodic. Because it was so highly valued for its ability to calm the central nervous system, it was even used to treat epilepsy. Europeans are well aware of its ability to induce sleep without the negative side effects of prescription hypnotic drugs. Ironically, unlike sleeping pills, Valerian Root has the ability to energize the body and the mind.[5] In Europe, Valerian is a popular, reliable and trusted sleep aid that is also used to calm nervous stomachs and relieve the symptoms of stress.

CHARACTER: nervine, sedative, carminative, and tonic

ACTIVE COMPOUNDS: It is the valpotriates, a group of chemical esters, which give Valerian Root its sedative properties. In addition, the valerenic and isovaleric acids contained in the herb also calm the central nervous system while relaxing smooth muscle.

MEDICINAL APPLICATIONS: insomnia, hyperexcitability, anxiety, tension, high blood pressure, stress, nervous stomach, palpitations, menstrual cramps, muscle spasms

SCIENTIFIC UPDATE: Volumes concerning the emerging value of Valerian Root as a natural calming agent could be compiled based on recent research findings. Clinical studies have found that Valerian tranquilizes and regulates the autonomic nervous system, enhances higher brain functions, and eases childhood psychosomatic disturbances and behavioral disorders.[6,7,8] A double blind study involving 128 subjects showed that Valerian improved sleep quality with none of the drawback of barbiturates.[9] Valerian actually reduced the morning sleepiness associated with sleeping aids. Valerian Root is also highly recommended for anyone who suffers from cardiovascular disease or hypertension in that it helps to relax smooth muscle and ease tension.

SAFETY: No known toxicity exists. Valerian is regarded as safe.[10] Extreme doses should be avoided. Pregnant women should consult their physician before taking Valerian. Because of its very pungent odor, the most palatable way to take Valerian Root is in capsulized form.

COMPLEMENTARY AGENTS: Hops, Chamomile, Passion Flower, Skullcap, Mullein, Marshmallow, Wood Betony, Hawthorne Berries, and Black Cohosh, Niacin, Calcium/Magnesium, Vitamin-B6, Melatonin

CHAMOMILE (MATRICARIA CHAMOMILLA)

OVERVIEW: For generations, Chamomile tea has been used as a favorite natural remedy to promote sleep and combat nervousness. Because it is relatively mild, it works best when combined with other nervine herbs. Chamomile has been described as a traditional "cure all" in that it has the ability to induce relaxation, prevent intestinal distress, including indigestion and heartburn and restore a sense of well being in the midst of upsetting situations. In addition, its bioflavonoid content makes it a good anti-inflammatory for conditions like arthritis. Its antiseptic properties favor its use for skin disorders.

CHARACTER: nervine, antispasmodic, anodyne, sedative, carminative, diaphoretic and tonic

ACTIVE COMPOUNDS: Flavonoids, (apigenine and luteoline), and Chamazulene and Alpha Bisabolol found in the volatile oil content of the flower, and dicyclic ether.

MEDICINAL APPLICATIONS: insomnia, anxiety, skin irritations, arthritis, menstrual cramps, and gastrointestinal distress.

SCIENTIFIC UPDATES: Recent studies have confirmed that Chamomile works as a uterine tonic, relaxes the nervous system, and interacts positively with other nervine herbs.[11] It has anti-bacterial properties, can stimulate the liver, and is currently under study for its anti-carcinogenic action.[12,13,14,15]

SAFETY: No toxicity has been found in Chamomile. Avoid extreme doses. Allergic reactions are rare.

COMPLEMENTARY AGENTS: Valerian Root, Skullcap, Hops, Wood Betony, Black Cohosh, Mullein, Marshmallow, Passion Flower, Peppermint, Vitamin B-complex, Vitamin C, Vitamin A, Calcium/Magnesium, Melatonin

SKULLCAP (SCUTELLARIA LATERIFLORA)

OVERVIEW: Skullcap had such a good reputation for its antispasmodic action that it was used in the 19th century to treat the symptoms of rabies.[16] Traditionally prescribed as a natural anti-convulsant by Native Americans, Europeans discovered its value for treating insomnia and even malaria. Today, Skullcap is considered one of the best herbs for treating a variety of nervous disorders. David Hoffman, in The Holistic Herbal refers to Skullcap as "the most widely relevant nervine available to us in the Materia Media." It is an herbal relaxant and restorative for the central nervous system and is an excellent tonic in cases of mental or physical exhaustion. When combined with Wood Betony, its calming effect is significantly enhanced.

CHARACTER: nervine, antipyretic, antispasmodic, sedative and tonic

ACTIVE COMPOUNDS: a flavonoid (scutellarin), iridoids, tannins, and volatile oil

MEDICINAL APPLICATIONS: muscles spasms, neuralgia, tension, hysteria, pain

SCIENTIFIC UPDATES: Skullcap continues to be used as a mild neural sedative which has the ability to relieve headaches and other related pain. Studies have shown that it can tranquilize a restless and excited nervous system.[17] In addition, nervous twitching and muscle spasms were also calmed by Skullcap[18,19,20] An added bonus of Skullcap is its ability to lower blood serum cholesterol and prevent high blood pressure.[21,22] One American doctor wrote, "Skullcap is a valuable tonic nervine and antispasmodic. It is especially useful in ...nervous excitability, restlessness, and inability to sleep..."[23]

SAFETY: Skullcap is considered safe when taken in appropriate dosages. One advantage of using Skullcap in an herbal blend is that its dose has been metered out in proportion with other herbs.

COMPLEMENTARY AGENTS: Valerian Root, Chamomile, Hops, Passion Flower, Wood Betony, Marshmallow, Mullein, Black Cohosh, B-complex, Folic Acid, Melatonin, Calcium/Magnesium

BLACK COHOSH (CIMICIFUGA RACEMOSA)

OVERVIEW: Black Cohosh has been used as a therapeutic botanical by Native Americans who harvested it in forests found in the Eastern U.S. and Canada. It was the herbal remedy of choice for mental and emotional disturbances which can accompany PMS and childbirth. While it works to balance hormones, it also exerts a calming and toning influence on the central nervous system. Black Cohosh tea is has been recommended for its sedating effect for generations. It is also a good source of calcium and magnesium which also tranquilize the nerves and prevent muscle cramping.

CHARACTER: sedative, diuretic, anti-inflammatory, anti-tussive, antispasmodic, alterative, emmenagogue

ACTIVE COMPOUNDS: alkaloids and glycosides

MEDICINAL APPLICATIONS: Black Cohosh has a number of desirable physiological benefits. Modern research has supported its use for hypertension and cardiovascular disorders.[24] While Black Cohosh can be used for ailments ranging from asthma to hormonal disruptions, its inclusion in this particular nervine formula hinge on its ability to tranquilize an irritable or excited nervous system while stimulating certain CNS functions which promote normalcy.

SCIENTIFIC UPDATES: Recently, the value of Black Cohosh as a uterine tonic has been supported by clinical research.[25] Current experimentation strongly suggests that Black Cohosh also has anti-inflammatory properties.[26,27,28,29] "Black Cohosh significantly relaxes nerves and smooth muscles and is effective in treating irritated nerves and general restlessness. The Russians have recently approved Black Cohosh extract for use as a central nervous system tonic and a treatment for high blood pressure."[30]

SAFETY: Black Cohosh is considered safe although pregnant women should consult their physician before using it. Avoid large doses.

COMPLEMENTARY AGENTS: Valerian Root, Hops, Wood Betony, Skullcap, Chamomile, Passion Flower, Mullein, Marshmallow, Melatonin, Calcium/Magnesium, B-complex

MARSHMALLOW (ALTHAEA OFFICINALIS)

OVERVIEW: Derived from the Greek word altho, meaning "to heal" Marshmallow has been used since before the time of ancient Egypt. It was one of the herbs found in the grave of a Neanderthal man.[31] The Marshmallow plant root contains the bulk of its medicinal properties. Its mucilaginous content has been traditionally used to coat, soothe and heal inflamed areas including respiratory, intestinal and urinary tissue. The calcium-rich content of Marshmallow contributes to its calming effect, however, its supportive role in soothing and healing inflamed mucous membranes is what makes it an effective anti-irritant.

CHARACTER: demulcent, emollient, expectorant, anti-inflammatory, diuretic, vulnerary

ACTIVE COMPOUNDS: mucilage, polysaccharides, asparagin, tannins

MEDICINAL APPLICATIONS: gastrointestinal upset, lung congestion, abrasions, dry coughs, sore throats, colitis, urinary tract infections, nervous exhaustion or breakdown

SCIENTIFIC UPDATES: Recent laboratory findings disclose that Marshmallow contains 286,000 units of vitamin A per pound which helps to boost its healing power.[32] The ability of Marshmallow to soothe and heal irritated respiratory passages is well documented.[33,34,35] It does the same for the gastro-intestinal system.[36]

SAFETY: Marshmallow is considered safe and non-toxic.

COMPLEMENTARY AGENTS: Black Cohosh, Burdock, Slippery Elm, Hops, Valerian Root, Skullcap, Mullein, Wood Betony, Chamomile, Melatonin, Vitamin E, Schizandra, Calcium/Magnesium, Inositol, Vitamin C, Vitamin A, and Niacin

WOOD BETONY (BETONICA OFFICINALIS)

OVERVIEW: Musa, an ancient Roman herbalist and physician to Caesar Augustus actually wrote an entire treatise on the merits of Wood Betony. It has good nervine properties for the reduction of nervousness through its mild sedative action. In medieval times, Wood Betony was one of the most highly prized herbs and was used to help normalize nervous disorders and ward off "ill humors." Today, the herb is used to encourage safe and restful sleep and to tone the glandular system. It is regarded as a favorite natural relaxant of Europeans and is also commonly used to treat headaches. It's vasodilator action has been scientifically documented.

CHARACTER: nervine, alterative, analgesic, hepatic, sedative, aromatic

ACTIVE COMPOUNDS: alkaloids (stachydrine, trigonelline), tannins, saponins

MEDICINAL APPLICATIONS: nervous disorders, headaches (especially tension), insomnia, hysteria, facial pain, liver protectant, Parkinson's disease

SCIENTIFIC UPDATES: Today, scientists have found that Wood Betony has the ability to dilate blood vessels and promote relaxation[37,38] This vascular effect has been linked to its ability to relieve headache pain, hence causing muscles to relax.[39]

SAFETY: Wood Betony is considered safe when taken in appropriate doses. Because it has the ability to mildly stimulate the uterus, it should be avoided in pregnancy.

COMPLEMENTARY AGENTS: Valerian, Hops, Skullcap, Marshmallow, Mullein, Chamomile, Black Cohosh, Melatonin, Lavender, Vitamin B-complex, and Calcium/Magnesium

MULLEIN (VERBASCUM THAPSUS)

OVERVIEW: Mullein is an impressive pain reliever that was used during the Civil War to treat respiratory infections. The pain relieving properties of Mullein are the result of its mild narcotic action which quiets agitated nerves while soothing inflammation. Mullein has traditionally been used to induce sleep in people suffering from nagging coughs, cramps or other spasms. Its high mucilage content makes it an effective cough and sore throat preparation

CHARACTER: sedative, demulcent, anti-spasmodic, antitussive, expectorant, analgesic, astringent, vulnerary

ACTIVE COMPOUNDS: mucilage, saponins, volatile oil, flavonoids, and bitter glycosides

MEDICINAL USES: colds, coughs, cramps, ear infections, insomnia, nervousness, respiratory problems, sore joints, pain

SCIENTIFIC UPDATES: Recent laboratory studies have found that the saponins and mucilage contained in Mullein enable it to heal and soothe inflammation.[40] In addition, testing concluded that Mullein can be used as an herbal pain reliever and sleep aid.[41]

SAFETY: Mullein is recognized as safe when used as recommended.

COMPLEMENTARY AGENTS: Marshmallow, Slippery Elm, Horehound, Hops, Skullcap, Valerian Root, Wood Betony, Black Cohosh, Lobelia, Melatonin, Vitamin C, Vitamin E, Calcium/Magnesium

THE GASTRO-INTESTINAL SYSTEM

DISORDERS TARGETED: indigestion, ulcers, flatulence, colitis, colic, heartburn, irritable bowel syndrome, nausea, bloating

Herbal Formula Two

Catnip, Myrrh Gum, Capsicum, Saw Palmetto, Peppermint, Calcium Carbonate

While many disorders of the G.I. tract are due to a poor diet that is usually low in fiber and high in sugar, fats and meat protein, some maladies come from life-style liabilities and stress. Nausea, heartburn and intestinal gas have made over-the-counter stomach remedies some of the most purchased medicines in the world. Gastric ulcers and a variety of bowel diseases plague great segments of our population and support the notion that we are not eating wisely. A good herbal formula designed to sustain and treat intestinal disorders must incorporate stimulating peristalsis, healing inflammation and inhibiting the formation of gas. Each individual function of the gastro-intestinal system must be supported and enhanced.

This formula does just that by bringing together herbs that have different functions which are amplified by their biochemical interaction.

*Catnip inhibits stomach spasms caused by gas and gently stimulates digestion.
*Myrrh Gum normalizes mucous membrane secretions in the stomach and protects against the formation of gastric ulcers.

*Capsicum stimulates digestion and helps to heal ulceration while expediting the medicinal effects of the other herbs it combines with.
*Saw Palmetto helps restore normal appetite and enhances nutrient assimilation while stimulating endocrine function.
*Peppermint works as an excellent carminative which relaxes the lower sphincter muscles of the esophagus easing heartburn and gas while strengthening and toning the stomach.

Individual Herbs

CATNIP (NEPETA CATARIA)

OVERVIEW: A member of the mint family, Europeans have used Catnip for centuries as a popular beverage tea. Native Americans found it effective for treating colic in infants. Catnip usually plays a supporting role in herbal combinations and is best known for its traditional use as an inhibitor of intestinal gas. Because it is a stomachic and antispasmodic, it can help to inhibit intestinal spasms and cramping caused by gas. It is soothing to the stomach and bowels and can also promote rest. In addition, Catnip was utilized for its ability to promote sweating in cases of colds and flu when fever is present. It is well suited to gastrointestinal disorders in that it inhibits gas formation, calms an upset stomach, aids digestion, and prevents and treats heartburn. Catnip is one of the most soothing carminatives found in the plant kingdom.
CHARACTER: antacid, antispasmodic, analgesic, carminative, emmenagogue, stomachic, diaphoretic, tonic
ACTIVE COMPOUNDS: Nepetalactones (volatile oils that absorb intestinal gas)
MEDICINAL APPLICATIONS: colic, intestinal gas, bloating, diarrhea, stomach cramping, insomnia, colds, flu, fevers, pain
SCIENTIFIC UPDATES: Today Catnip is sometimes called " Nature's Alka Seltzer" due to its ability to stimulate digestion.[42] It also has some antibiotic properties which may help to control stomach bacteria.[43] It is used for a wide variety of ailments including insomnia, and anemia and is rich in organic iron, which helps to build the blood.
SAFETY: Catnip is considered a safe botanical medicine if used appropriately.
COMPLEMENTARY AGENTS: Ginger, Fennel, Peppermint, Papaya, Capsicum, Saw Palmetto Berry, Myrrh Gum, Calcium Carbonate, Pepsin, Acidophilus

MYRRH GUM (COMMIPHORA MOLMOL)

OVERVIEW: Myrrh is extracted from a resin that is collected from bushy shrubs native to Arabia and Somalia, and has been esteemed as an Eastern herbal treasure for thousands of years. Brought to fame through its reference in the Bible as one of the gifts of the magi, Myrrh was used to honor births and to anoint the dead. Ancient Egyptians used to burn Myrrh as incense to fumigate their homes. While Myrrh works as a disinfectant within the urinary tract, it also expedites the removal of excess mucus. Regarding the gastrointestinal system, Myrrh acts to directly stimulate the peptic glands which increases digestive activity and efficiency. Sometimes, poor digestion is due to excess mucus formation in the stomach and intestines.

CHARACTER: astringent, antiseptic, antibacterial, expectorant, hepato-protective, carminative, tonic

ACTIVE COMPOUNDS: volatile oils (limonene, eugenol, pinene), resins and gums

MEDICINAL APPLICATIONS: congestion, indigestion, gas, ulcers, irritable bowel syndrome, ulcerative colitis, diverticulitis, Crohn's disease, wound healing, sore throats, gingivitis

SCIENTIFIC UPDATES: Myrrh normalized mucous membrane activity.[44] Because the mucous lining of the stomach is so important for its protection from stomach acids, Myrrh is considered a valuable digestive aid. In addition, if too much mucus is secreted in the gastrointestinal tract, digestion in impaired. Myrrh helps to ensure the proper function of mucous secreting glands and exerts an antiseptic and antibacterial action at the same time.[45]

SAFETY: Myrrh has a mild uterine stimulant action and should be avoided in pregnancy.

COMPLEMENTARY AGENTS: Ginger, Fenugreek, Catnip, Peppermint, Fennel, Capsicum, Acidophilus, Saw Palmetto, Slippery Elm, Calcium/Magnesium, Vitamin A, Vitamin B-Complex, Vitamin E, and Digestive Enzymes

CAPSICUM (CAPSICUM ANNUM)

OVERVIEW: Capsicum, also known as cayenne pepper, was first introduced to Europe after Columbus returned from the New World. Known as the "plant with a bite," Capsicum has a variety of uses both therapeutically and as a popular culinary spice. Commonly used for throat and skin infections, Capsicum became a favorite of 19th-century physiomedicalists who prescribed it for rheumatism and depression. Capsicum has the ability to stimulate and heal. It has been used to initiate the flow of mucus making it a valuable treatment for respiratory disorders. Its addition to herbal blends is also based on the fact that it can dramatically increase the efficiency of other herbs it combines with.

CHARACTER: gastric stimulant, antiseptic, antibacterial, carminative, diaphoretic, tonic

ACTIVE COMPOUNDS: capsaicin (what makes it hot), carotenoids, flavonoids, volatile oils

MEDICINAL APPLICATIONS: arthritis, bronchitis, colds, fatigue, respiratory disorders, fevers, tonsillitis, hoarseness, migraines, obesity, circulatory disorders, indigestion, lack of appetite, ulcers

SCIENTIFIC UPDATES: Capsicum enables ingested foods to be better assimilated.[46] It's stimulatory action boosts circulation and saliva production which inevitably results in better digestion.[47] It also increases perspiration helping to remove toxins in the blood. Capsicum is a multifaceted herb which can inhibit the formation of gas, and GI tract spasms while promoting the coagulation of blood.[48] For this reason, it has been used to prevent external and internal hemorrhaging. Clinical studies have also documented the ability of Capsicum to stimulate the heart and to lower blood serum cholesterol.[49] Additional studies have indicated the Capsicum has the ability to slow fat absorption in the small intestines and increase the metabolic rate (thermogenesis).[50]

SAFETY: If pregnant or nursing, check with your physician before using. Avoid contact with the eyes and use in recommended dosages only.

COMPLEMENTARY AGENTS: Peppermint, Garlic, Ginger, Fennel, Saw Palmetto, Catnip, Myrrh, Vitamin C, Vitamin A

SAW PALMETTO (SERENOA REPENS)

OVERVIEW: Considered an old Native American tonic, Saw Palmetto dates back to the ancient Mayan civilization. This herb was traditionally used to stimulate the appetite encouraging normal weight gain in debilitated conditions. It is considered a general tonic which nourishes the body with specific emphasis on the mucous membranes and hormonal tissue. Used for treating male and female genito-urinary ailments, it acquired an impressive reputation for relieving bladder obstructions caused by an enlarged prostate gland.

CHARACTER: anti-catarrhal, anti-inflammatory, antiseptic, anti-spasmodic, diuretic, expectorant, hormonal, nutritive, stimulant, tonic

ACTIVE COMPOUNDS: steroidal saponins, fatty acids, volatile oil, phytosterols, resin, tannins, polysaccharides

MEDICINAL APPLICATIONS: prostate disease, genito-urinary problems, endocrine disorders, infertility, impotence, bronchitis, colds, menstrual disorders, ovarian dysfunction, lactation, thyroid deficiencies, digestive problems, painful periods

SCIENTIFIC UPDATES: The ability of Saw Palmetto to treat Prostate disease has been the subject of recent clinical studies. The results have been impressive and strongly suggest that Saw Palmetto may be a viable alternative to the use of Proscar, a pharmaceutical drug used for treating enlarged Prostate glands.[51] Its inclusion in digestive formulas is based on its ability to stimulate normal appetite and boost nutrient assimilation.[52] Saw Palmetto may also be useful for women who suffer from hormonal imbalances by helping to normalize estrogen levels.

SAFETY: No toxicity has been reported with Saw Palmetto

COMPLEMENTARY AGENTS: B-Complex, Calcium/Magnesium, Calcium Carbonate, Ginger, Proanthocyanidins, Phytonutrients, Bee Pollen, Fennel, Catnip, Peppermint, Capsicum, Acidophilus, Kelp, Sarsaparilla, Ginseng, Digestive Enzymes, Bee Pollen, Bee Propolis

PEPPERMINT (MENTHA PIPERITA)

OVERVIEW: Peppermint is an old tried and true remedy and has been used for centuries to treat digestive and bowel disorders. Chinese and Greek medical records support its use since 659 A.D. for everything from hiccups to dog bites. Today, it is prescribed as a stomach relaxant that helps to eliminate the formation of gas and griping pain. It is frequently combined with other herbs to facilitate better digestion. Its inclusion in colon cleansing and gastro-intestinal tonics is more than justified due to its stomach action. It is also important to know that the stimulatory properties of Peppermint enhance the action of other herbs it combines with.

CHARACTER: anti-spasmodic, anti-nauseate, analgesic, aromatic, astringent, calmative, carminative, choleretic, diaphoretic, digestive stimulant, nervine, sedative, stomachic, tonic

ACTIVE COMPOUNDS: leaf and distilled volatile oils (menthol), tannins, flavonoids, tocopherols, choline

MEDICINAL APPLICATIONS: colds, sinusitis, bronchitis, diarrhea, gastritis, enteritis, indigestion, nausea, gas, bloating, gripping, colic, colitis, heartburn, irritable bowel syndrome, gallstones, stomach spasms, ulcers, vomiting

SCIENTIFIC UPDATES: Today, Peppermint is recognized for its soothing action on the stomach and intestines. It works as an ant-spasmodic which helps to relieve nausea, and other stomach maladies. Peppermint relaxes the muscles of the digestive tract and stimulates bile flow, which facilitates more efficient digestion.[53] Increased bile flow results in less indigestion, flatulence and colic.[54] The menthol constituent of Peppermint works as a natural analgesic and antibacterial.[55] One of the primary reasons Peppermint is considered such an excellent digestive aid that it acts in two separate ways to normalize gastrointestinal activity. First, it stimulates gallbladder activity, and secondly, it absorbs intestinal gas and eases stomach cramping.[56] In addition, Peppermint has demonstrated anti-ulcer, anti-inflammatory and anti-bacterial actions, all of which contribute to its use as an overall therapeutic botanical.[57] Peppermint has also been able to dissolve gallstones and may be a nonsurgical approach to gallstone removal.[58]

SAFETY: When used in normal and appropriate dosages, Peppermint is considered quite safe. Oil of Peppermint can be irritating to mucous membranes if used excessively. Use with caution if pregnant or breast-feeding.

COMPLEMENTARY AGENTS: Catnip, Fennel, Ginger, Myrrh, Capsicum, Saw Palmetto, Calcium Carbonate, Digestive Enzymes

NOTE: The addition of calcium in carbonate form makes it easily absorbable and contributes to better digestion by preventing heartburn and by absorbing excess stomach acid.

COLON CLEANSER

DISORDERS TARGETED: Congestion, Crohn's Disease, Colitis, Constipation, Diarrhea, Diverticulitis, Irritable Bowel Syndrome, Gallbladder Disease, Hemorrhoids, Liver Disorders, Parasites, Worms,

Herbal Formula Three

Cascara Sagrada, Black Walnut, Buckthorn, Couch Grass, Culver Root, Pumpkin Seeds, Quassia, Red Clover, Garlic

The purpose of this blend is to provide nutritive support while stimulating intestinal cleansing and detoxification. Ridding the intestines of parasites, cleansing the blood and strengthening the liver and gallbladder are also involved in optimal colon cleansing. Frequently, seemingly unrelated health problems can be traced to a sluggish or congested colon. Harboring toxic waste in the large intestine can pose a significant health risk, Carcinogens, altered hormones and other poisonous chemical compounds can be reabsorbed into the body if not eliminated properly. In addition, disorders like chronic constipation attest to poor dietary habits and a lack of colonic health. These herbs provide the optimal blend for colon function which will, inevitably, improve overall health.

*Cascara Sagrada gently promotes colon evacuation while providing tone to colonic muscle.
*Black Walnut assists intestinal detoxification by killing parasites and worms.
*Buckthorn contains aloe emodin, which stimulate peristalsis and mucous secretion thereby facilitating the expulsion of toxic waste from the intestines.
*Couch Grass acts as a blood purifier and exerts a natural antibiotic action on a variety of bacteria and molds.
*Culver Root effectively removes old debris from the bowels, purifies the blood and promotes better digestion.
*Pumpkin Seeds assist Black Walnut in killing intestinal parasites while stimulating the prostate gland.
*Quassia also facilitates the expulsion of intestinal worms and toxic waste due to improper digestion.
*Red Clover efficiently clears the blood of toxins and helps the intestines to discharge nitrogenous waste.
*Garlic's multifaceted properties kill parasites, worms, bacteria, viruses, lower cholesterol, and stimulate the lymphatic system to throw off waste material.

Individual Herbs

CASCARA SAGRADA (RHAMNUSD PURSHIANA)

OVERVIEW: Known as "sacred bark" Cascara Sagrada has been used as a reliable and safe natural laxative for generations. Cascara has the remarkable ability to promote regularity without addiction or gripping typical of other laxative agents. It has also been reported to tonify the bowel, which means that its beneficial effects continue after the herb is no longer taken. Several over-the-counter preparations use Cascara but sometimes combine it with harsher synthetic chemicals. It is an excellent addition to any intestinal cleanser herbal preparation.

CHARACTER: anti-bacterial, anti-parasitic, cathartic, emetic, hepato-tonic, laxative, purgative, cholagogue,

ACTIVE COMPOUNDS: Hydroxy anthracene derivatives (HAD), free anthraquinone glycosides (emodin, frangulin, isoemodin, aloe-emodin, chrysophanol), rhein, aloins

MEDICINAL APPLICATIONS: congestion (general), constipation, colon disorders (sluggish colon etc), gallbladder disease, gallstones, gas, hemorrhoids, jaundice, kidney stone prevention, liver disorders, parasites, worms

SCIENTIFIC UPDATES: The aloe-emodin content of Cascara has shown antileukemic properties.[59] The anthraquinones have exhibited potent antibacterial properties against intestinal bacteria.[60] The rhein content of Cascara is used in Africa to expel worms.[61] Cascara increases muscular activity in the large intestine.[62] Cascara can prevent the occurrence of calcium based urinary stones.[63] "Cascara is perhaps the safest and most certain laxative available and can be used to restore tone to the colon and thereby overcome laxative dependency in the elderly. The herb is safe and effective for detoxification and cleansing programs..."[64]

SAFETY: At recommended dosages, no toxicity. Cascara should not be used by nursing mothers as its laxative effect can transfer to infant. Pregnant women should avoid using Cascara unless directed by their doctor to do so. People with ulcers or irritable bowel syndrome should check with their doctor before using Cascara Sagrada.

COMPLEMENTARY AGENTS: Dandelion, Black Walnut, Quassia, Red Clover, Garlic, Buckthorn, Pumpkin Seeds, Marshmallow, Slippery Elm, Culver Root, Acidophilus, Vitamin A, B-complex, Vitamin E, Calcium/Magnesium

BLACK WALNUT (JUGLANS NIGRA)

OVERVIEW: Europeans have turned to Black Walnut for its ability to act as an intestinal tonic and to treat skin disorders. During the Civil War, it was prescribed for diarrhea and dysentery. Black Walnut has the ability to kill parasites and fungal infections without posing a risk to healthy tissue.

CHARACTER: anthelmintic, antifungal, antiparasitic, antiseptic, antispasmodic, astringent, digestive tonic, insecticide, laxative

ACTIVE COMPOUNDS: quinones, oils, tannins

MEDICINAL APPLICATIONS: athlete's foot, boils, Candida albicans (yeast infections), canker sores, cold sores, eczema, fungus, gum disease, herpes, intestinal parasites, tapeworm, tuberculosis

SCIENTIFIC UPDATES: Recent research strongly suggests that Black Walnut has antifungal properties as well as an antiseptic action.[65] Clinical studies have found that certain constituents in Black Walnut have anti-cancer properties.[66] The high tannin content of Black Walnut is primarily responsible for it ability to expel worms and parasites.[67] "Black Walnut has been shown to be specific for treatment of Candida albicans."[68]

SAFETY: Use in appropriate amounts as directed. Pregnant or nursing mothers should check with their physicians.

COMPLEMENTARY AGENTS: Garlic, Cascara Sagrada, Buckthorn, Pumpkin Seeds, Red Clover, Culver Root, Acidophilus, Vitamin A, B-complex, Pantothenic Acid, Calcium/Magnesium, Potassium, Marine Lipids

BUCKTHORN (RHAMNUS FRANGULA)

OVERVIEW: As early as the second century A.D., Galen, the Greek Physician wrote about the merits of Buckthorn. On this continent, Native Americans used Buckthorn as a cathartic and skin remedy. Buckthorn is similar to Cascara Sagrada in its ability to gently ease constipation and stimulate the normal evacuation of the bowels. As a hot tea, Buckthorn can also promote perspiration and help lower fever. It is also considered a liver and gallbladder tonic.

CHARACTER: alterative, anthelmintic, cathartic, depurative, emetic, laxative

ACTIVE COMPOUNDS: anthraquinones glycosides

MEDICINAL APPLICATIONS: bowel cleansing, cancer, constipation, fever, gallbladder disease, gallstones, liver ailments

SCIENTIFIC UPDATES: Buckthorn has shown significant inhibition of leukemia in mice studies.[69] Buckthorn contains anthraquinone glycosides which works like Cascara Sagrada to promote gentle colon peristalsis.[70] European studies have confirmed that advantage of Buckthorn's ability to release its active principles in the small intestine rather than the stomach.[71]

SAFETY: Take as directed in appropriate doses. Pregnant or nursing women should avoid this herb due to its laxative effect.

COMPLEMENTARY AGENTS: Cascara Sagrada, Red Clover, Pumpkin Seeds, Culver Root, Marshmallow, Slippery Elm, Dandelion, Black Walnut, Quassia, Ginger, Acidophilus, Vitamin A, Vitamin E, B-complex, Bioflavonoids, Marine Lipids

COUCH GRASS (AGROPYRON REPENS)

OVERVIEW: Couch Grass has traditionally been used to treat urinary tract infections due to its soothing demulcent properties. The roots of Couch Grass are considered a wholesome food for cattle and horses. The diuretic action of thisherb helps to promote urine flow thereby cleansing the blood of toxins. Its ability to act as a purgative and purify the blood of poisons makes it a good addition to any cleansing formula.

CHARACTER: antibiotic, demulcent, depurative, diuretic, emollient, pectoral, tonic

ACTIVE COMPOUNDS: triticin, mucilage, acid malates, inocite

MEDICINAL APPLICATIONS: bladder infections, blood purifier, jaundice, kidney disease, rheumatism

SCIENTIFIC UPDATES: Extracts of Couch Grass have exhibited antibiotic effects on a variety of bacteria and molds.[72] Couch Grass has been known to eliminate kidney stones.[73]

SAFETY: Take in appropriate doses as recommended. An excess could lead to potassium and other mineral deficiency.

COMPLEMENTARY AGENTS: Uva Ursi, Cornsilk, Parsley, Juniper, Cascara Sagrada, Red Clover, Garlic, Black Walnut, Vitamin C, Bioflavonoids, Vitamin A, Vitamin E, Potassium, Magnesium, Copper, Mineral and Electrolyte Supplements

CULVER ROOT (VERONICASTRUM VIRGINCUM)

OVERVIEW: It was Dr. Culver who introduced this root from Native American Indians to the white community. It is considered a stomach tonic and can help to remove intestinal waste matter in a mild way. Culver Root nicely complements other laxative herbs and like Cascara and Buckthorn, and does not have the negative side effects of other intestinal purgatives.

CHARACTER: alterative, blood purifier, cathartic, cholagogue, emetic, purgative, hepatic, laxative, tonic

ACTIVE COMPOUNDS: volatile oil, tannic acid, gum, resin, leptandrin, ester of p-methoxycinnamic acid, phytosterol verosterol

MEDICINAL APPLICATIONS: blood purifier, constipation, diarrhea, colon congestion, liver ailments, stomach disorders

SCIENTIFIC UPDATES: Culver's Root works chiefly on the intestines in chronic constipation due to poor biliary flow. It has a mild action without causing the depression of physical strength common with many other purgative medicines."[74] "Leptandrin excites the liver gently and promotes the secretion of bile without irritating the bowels."[75]

SAFETY: Pregnant or Nursing mothers should not take this herb without their doctor's consent.

COMPLEMENTARY AGENTS: Buckthorn, Cascara Sagrada, Red Raspberry, Ginger, Fennel, Black Walnut, Quassia, Garlic, Couch Grass, Acidophilus, Vitamin C, Bioflavonoids, Vitamin A, B-complex, Marine Lipids, Phytonutrients, Blue-Green Algae

PUMPKIN SEED (CUCURBITA PEPO)

OVERVIEW: Pumpkin Seed has been used for generations as a natural diuretic, to kill intestinal parasites and to revitalize the prostate gland. The pulverized seed has been used as a treatment for tapeworm and roundworm. In addition, Pumpkin Seed has the ability to act as a mild diuretic and to alleviate nausea.
CHARACTER: demulcent, diuretic, laxative, nutritive, parasiticide
ACTIVE COMPOUNDS: fixed oil, volatile oil, acrid resin, myocin
MEDICINAL APPLICATIONS: prostate disorders, intestinal parasites
SCIENTIFIC UPDATES: Recent Swedish clinical trials found the that oil constituents of pumpkin seed combined with Saw Palmetto effectively treated an enlarged prostate gland.[76] "Pumpkin Seed has a reputation of being a non-irritating diuretic."[77] Pumpkin Seed contains a rare amino acid called myocin found in the seeds of certain Cucurbita species which is the primary protein constituent of muscles.[78]
SAFETY: Take as directed.
COMPLEMENTARY AGENTS: Saw Palmetto, Kelp, Garlic, Black Walnut, Red Clover, Cascara Sagrada, Quassia, Buckthorn, Acidophilus, Bee Pollen, Bee Propolis, B-complex, Vitamin E, Bioflavonoids, Phytonutrients, Blue/Green Algae, Zinc, Electrolyte Supplements

QUASSIA (PICRASMA AMARA)

OVERVIEW: Native to Jamaica, Quassia can be found in various forms throughout local herb shops. Used to kill worms and to stimulate the appetite after a debilitating disease, Quassia has powerful medicinal properties. It has been aptly referred to as a great healer of the sick. Used as an overall tonic, it has the reputation of destroying one's taste for alcoholic beverages.
CHARACTER: antispasmodic, bitter tonic, stomachic, vermicide, hepatotonic
ACTIVE COMPOUNDS: volatile oil, quassin, gummy extractive pectin, tartrate, sulphate of lime, calcium chlorides
MEDICINAL APPLICATIONS: anorexia, convalescence, elderly emaciation, indigestion, fever, worms

SCIENTIFIC UPDATES: Quassia lessens putrefaction in the stomach, and prevents the formation of acid substances during digestion.[79] It is said to be one of the best remedies of noxious substances in the alimentary canal resulting from inadequate digestion.[80]

SAFETY: Because of its potency, it is better to take Quassia in herbal formulations than alone to avoid stomach irritation and nausea.

COMPLEMENTARY AGENTS: Black Walnut, Cascara Sagrada, Garlic, Buckthorn, Ginger, Pumpkin Seed, Red Clover, Peppermint, Vitamin E, Vitamin C, Bioflavonoids, Proanthocyanidins, B-complex Acidophilus, Phytonutrients, Blue/Green Algae

RED CLOVER (TRIFOLIUM PRATENSE)

OVERVIEW: Originally Red Clover was used to feed cattle. Medieval Christians associated its three-leafed configuration with the Trinity, and the Romans prescribed it for kidney stones. Its medicinal use today is based on its impressive ability to clear the body of mucus and other toxins. Because it can purify the blood, it is an excellent therapeutic herb for skin disorders. For over a century, it has been used to treat and prevent cancer.

CHARACTER: alterative, anti-inflammatory, antispasmodic, anti-cancer, diuretic, possible estrogenic

ACTIVE COMPOUNDS: phenolic glycosides, flavonoids, salicylates, coumarins, cyanogenic glycosides, mineral acids

MEDICINAL APPLICATIONS: acne, bladder infections, blood cleanser, boils, bronchitis, cancer, leukemia, liver disorders, nervous conditions, psoriasis, skin ailments, tumors

SCIENTIFIC UPDATES: Clinical studies have found that Red Clover contains antibiotic properties against several bacteria including those that cause tuberculosis.[81] Scientists have discovered that Red Clover contains molybdenum, a trace element that is now recognized as essential in clearing the body of nitrogenous waste material.[82] "Many naturopathic physicians use the herb as an alterative including it in regular cleansing programs."[83]

SAFETY: Take as directed. No known toxicity.

COMPLEMENTARY AGENTS: Licorice, Buckthorn, Cascara Sagrada, Sarsaparilla, Alfalfa, Quassia, Black Walnut, Kelp, Blue/Green Algae, Phytonutrients, Vitamin C, Bioflavonoids, Acidophilus

GARLIC (ALLIVUM SATIVUM)

OVERVIEW: Garlic has graced the pages of ancient records since history was recorded and is nothing less than remarkable in its curative properties. For centuries, an impressive array of medicinal powers have been attributed to this botanical. Ancient Egyptians, Greeks and Romans turned to Garlic for everything from fighting infection to warding off evil spirits. Early in the twentieth century, Garlic was used therapeutically to treat tuberculosis and to fight infection from war wounds. Pasteur scientifically proved that Garlic is a powerful antibiotic and today, modern clinicians and researchers are beginning to uncover the marvelous healing properties of Garlic in the laboratory.

CHARACTER: alterative, antibiotic, anti-cancer, antifungal, antiviral, anti-Candida, antiparasitic, anti-worm, anti-protozoan, anti-toxin, aromatic, carminative, diaphoretic, diuretic, digestive tonic, expectorant, immunostimulant, stomachic, tonic

ACTIVE COMPOUNDS: alliin, allinase, allicin

MEDICINAL APPLICATIONS: arteriosclerosis, arthritis, asthma, blood poisoning, blood pressure (high or low), bronchitis, cancer, Candida, circulatory insufficiency, colds, colitis, coughs, digestive disorders, ear infections, fever, flu, fungus, gas, heart disease, infections (viral and bacterial), liver ailments, lung disorders, parasites, pinworm, prostate gland disorders, respiratory congestion, yeast infections

SCIENTIFIC UPDATES: Garlic has been the subject of intense scientific study over the last three decades. Recent research has proven the value of Garlic in treating and preventing cardiovascular disease. Controlled studies discovered that it can lower cholesterol and triglyceride levels, reduce the tendency of the blood to clot, and decrease blood pressure.[84] Garlic has scientifically proven its ability to inhibit bacterial growth.[85] One milligram of allicin, Garlic's primary constituent, is estimated to equal 15 standard units of penicillin.[86] Dr. Erik Block discovered that Garlic also protects the liver from drug, radiation and free radical damage.[87] Garlic can also stimulate immunity and is considered an anti-cancer agent.[88]

SAFETY: Garlic is considered safe, however, an excess dose can cause stomach upset. When using Garlic directly on the skin, coat the area with olive oil first to avoid skin irritation. Do not use Garlic in large amounts if you have anemia or ulcers.

COMPLEMENTARY AGENTS: Parsley, Capsicum, Alfalfa, Blue/Green Algae, Kelp, Black Walnut, Buckthorn, Couch Grass, Red Clover, Golden Seal, Vitamin C, Bioflavonoids, Proanthocyanidins, Phytonutrients

SYSTEMIC CLEANSER FOR INTERNAL ORGANS (COLON, LIVER, KIDNEYS AND LYMPH GLANDS)

Herbal Formula Four

Red Sage, Yellow Dock, Dandelion, Garlic, Cornsilk, Fenugreek, Quassia, Black Cohosh, Cascara Sagrada

Blood is the medium which carries oxygen and supplies nutrients to the vast cellular network of our bodies. Unfortunately, toxins and poisons can also circulate through the blood and must be filtered and removed by certain organ systems. This formula combines some of the most effective colon cleansers, liver tonics, and blood purifiers available. The blend provides nutritive and therapeutic support to the body and is ideal for anyone suffering from chronic disease or disability. In order to cleanse the liver, kidneys and the lymph, the blood must be filtered and cleared of carcinogens, chemicals, altered hormonal compounds, nitrogenous waste, allergens and a whole host of environmental pollutants.

* Red Sage acts as a high mineral tonic herb to promote an overall cleanse and stimulate bile flow for enhanced liver function.
*Yellow Dock boosts the livers ability to filter and purify the blood.
*Dandelion effectively clears toxins out of the bloodstream and promotes liver function even when the liver is compromised.
*Garlic stimulates the immune system to fight off infection and activates the lymph glands to more efficiently throw off waste materials.
*Cornsilk assists the kidneys in filtering uric acid by acting as an effective diuretic.
*Fenugreek absorbs bile acids and helps expel toxic waste and mucus through the channels of elimination.
*Quassia facilitates the removal of colon debris and helps to prevent autointoxication.
*Black Cohosh stimulates liver, kidney and lymph secretions.

*Cascara Sagrada acts as a liver tonic and promotes normal bowel evacuation preventing toxin re-entry into the bloodstream

Individual Herbs

RED SAGE (SALVIA OFFICINALIS)

OVERVIEW: Red Sage is another botanical that has a long history of use. Traditionally linked to longevity and mental alertness, Red Sage was also utilized for increased wisdom. Among its myriad of uses, Red Sage has been used for hot flashes, nervousness, and depression. It also acts as an overall tonic stimulating better liver function.

CHARACTER: antispasmodic, antiparasitic, antipyretic, antiseptic, aromatic, astringent, carminative, promotes bile flow, reduces blood sugar, tonic (overall)

ACTIVE COMPOUNDS: volatile oil, diterpene bitters, tannins, triterpenoids, resin, flavonoids, estrogenic agents, saponins

MEDICINAL APPLICATIONS: coughs, depression, diabetes, digestive disorders, fever, liver aliments, memory (failing), mouth sores, nausea, nervous conditions, nigh sweats, sores, sore throat, worms

SCIENTIFIC UPDATES: The volatile oils and tannins in Red Sage are responsible for its ability to stop excessive perspiration. The oils also have an antiseptic and astringent property which makes them useful in the healing of sores and irritations.[89] Red Sage also acts as a powerful antioxidant and boosts circulation.

SAFETY: Avoid medicinal dosages in pregnancy and in cases of epilepsy. Nursing mothers should not take Red Sage due to its milk drying action.

COMPLEMENTARY AGENTS: Capsicum, Dandelion, Garlic, Yellow Dock, Quassia, Milk Thistle, Cascara Sagrada, Black Walnut, Acidophilus, Blue/Green Algae, Phytonutrients, Proanthocyanidins, Vitamin C, Vitamin A, B-complex, Calcium/Magnesium

YELLOW DOCK (RUMEX CRISPUS)

OVERVIEW: A favorite among Native Americans, Yellow Dock was used for a variety of ailments with particular emphasis on skin eruptions. American herbalists subsequently used Yellow Dock for blood and glandular disorders including cancer. Today, the herb is considered one of the best botanical blood builders and is recommended for anemia, liver congestion and skin problems.

It remains the favorite alterative (blood purifier) of many different cultures. Its rich iron content makes it a valuable therapeutic agent for anemic conditions. It plays an integral role in any cleansing formula.

CHARACTER: alterative, astringent, cathartic, depurative, hepatic, laxative, nutritive (leaves), tonic

ACTIVE COMPOUNDS: rumicin, chrysarobin

MEDICINAL APPLICATIONS: anemia, blood disorders, blood cleanser, boils, cancer, coughs, hives, iron deficiency, liver ailments, psoriasis, rheumatism, skin disorders, sores

SCIENTIFIC UPDATES: Yellow Dock enhances the liver's ability to filter the blood.[91] Antibacterial properties have also been observed in Yellow Dock.[92] "Yellow Dock Root achieves its tonic properties through astringent purification of the blood supply to the glands...It is often used in seasonal cleanses and blood detoxification programs. Among all herbs, it has one of the strongest reputations for clearing up skin problems, liver and gallbladder ailments, and glandular inflammation and swelling.[93] Yellow Dock is considered an excellent lymphatic cleanser.

SAFETY: Use as directed.

COMPLEMENTARY AGENTS: Dandelion, Capsicum, Burdock, Garlic, Fenugreek, Quassia, Kelp, Black Cohosh, Red Sage, Blue/Green Algae, Vitamin C, Vitamin A, Bioflavonoids, B-complex, Proanthocyanidins, Phytonutrients

DANDELION (TARAXACUM OFFICINALE)

OVERVIEW: Dandelion is a relatively new herb not appearing in Chinese herbal records until the 7th century. Its name was the result of its lion-tooth shaped leaves. Dandelion is a potassium rich plant which has been used for a number of ailments throughout the world. Its strength lies in its inherent diuretic and liver enhancing properties. Dandelion has the ability to stimulate and detoxify liver tissue while promoting healthy, pure blood.

CHARACTER: antirheumatic, blood purifier, diuretic, hepato-tonic, laxative, nutritive, stomachic, tonic (general)

ACTIVE COMPOUNDS: bitter glycosides, tannins, triterpenes, sterols, volatile oil, choline, asparagine, inulin

MEDICINAL APPLICATIONS: acne, anemia, arthritis, asthma, blood disorders, eczema, gallbladder disease, hepatitis, hypoglycemia, jaundice, kidney infections, liver disorders, psoriasis, PMS, skin eruptions, weight loss

SCIENTIFIC UPDATES: Several clinical studies have supported the ability of

Dandelion to treat chronic liver congestion.[95] Dandelion has an impressive bile-stimulating action which helps promote liver and gallbladder function.[96] The ability of Dandelion to clear the gallbladder and treat jaundice has been impressive.[97] Modern research has proven the validity of Dandelion. It can stimulate the elimination of uric acid from the body and treat anemic conditions of the blood.[98]

SAFETY: Use as directed in appropriate doses.

COMPLEMENTARY AGENTS : Milk Thistle, Burdock, Yellow Dock, Cascara Sagrada, Fenugreek, Garlic, Red Sage, Red Clover, Black Cohosh, Vitamin C, Bioflavonoids, Proanthocyanidins, Vitamin A, B-Complex, Vitamin E, Phytonutrients, Blue/Green Algae

FENUGREEK (TRIGONELLA FOENUM-GRAECUM)

OVERVIEW: Fenugreek was a favorite therapeutic herb of Hippocrates, the Father of Medicine and is one of the oldest known medicinal herbs. Anciently, it was used to ensure easier childbirth, increase lactation, and ease menstrual pain. The Chinese have used it to treat gastric upsets and male impotence. Today, its value for blood sugar disorders is emerging. It has the ability to move mucus out of congested areas of the body. Fenugreek has been shown to expel mucus and toxic waste by way of the lymphatic system, making it a natural addition to cleansing herbal blends.

CHARACTER: alterative, anti-inflammatory, aphrodisiac, aromatic, astringent, carminative, demulcent, emollient, expectorant, hormonal, mucilant, nutritive, parasiticide, stomachic, tonic

ACTIVE COMPOUNDS: steroid saponins, alkaloids (trigonelline, gentianeine), mucilage

MEDICINAL APPLICATIONS: allergies, bronchitis, cholesterol levels, coughs, diabetes, digestive ailments, emphysema, intestinal gas, headache, lung infections, mucus congestion, skin eruptions

SCIENTIFIC UPDATES: Fenugreek is currently being used to treat diabetes in Middle East Countries.[99] Because it contains up to 30% mucilage, Fenugreek works as an effective anti-inflammatory agent and can heal abscesses and other skin eruptions. Clinical tests have shown that Fenugreek significantly reduced blood glucose and cholesterol levels in test animals.[100] Fenugreek seeds, which contain diosgenin and tigogenin may also help tone uterine muscle and stimulate lactation in nursing mothers.[101] French scientists have found that Fenugreek stimulates pancreatic secretion which enhances digestion.[102]

SAFETY: Fenugreek should be avoided in pregnancy as it is a uterine stimulant. Diabetics should check with their doctor's before using Fenugreek for blood sugar control.

COMPLEMENTARY AGENTS: Dandelion, Myrrh, Red Clover, Lobelia, Cornsilk, Garlic, Yellow Dock, Golden Seal, Vitamin C, Bioflavonoids, Proanthocyanidins, Phytonutrients, Blue/Green Algae, Vitamin A, B-Complex, Chromium

CORNSILK (ZEA MAYS)

OVERVIEW: Cornsilk was a favorite natural remedy for disorders of the genitourinary tract by Indians native to Central America. Its ability to heal irritated mucous membrane and act as an effective diuretic make it an ideal treatment for bladder and kidney related problems. For over a century it has been prescribed for bladder inflammations and enlarged prostate glands.

CHARACTER: alterative, diuretic, demulcent, lithotriptic

ACTIVE COMPOUNDS: maizenic acid, fatty acids, menthol, glycosides, thymol, saponins

MEDICINAL APPLICATIONS: albuminuria, bladder infections, edema, heart trouble, hepatitis, kidney disorders, prostatitis, urinary tract infections, water retention

SCIENTIFIC UPDATES: The maizenic acid contained in Cornsilk is responsible for its stimulating diuretic effect. In addition, this compound also benefits the liver and intestines and is considered a "cardiac solution" for the heart.[147] Clinical studies in China and Japan have demonstrated the remarkable diuretic properties of Cornsilk.[148]

" . . . Cornsilk directly reduces painful symptoms and swelling due to several inflammatory conditions including cystitis, pyelitis, oligouria, hepatitis and all edematous conditions."[149] In China it is also used for hypertension and diabetes.[150]

SAFETY: Take in appropriate doses as directed. Any substance that acts as a diuretic may cause a potassium deficiency if used in excess. Use potassium supplementation. Cornsilk is considered a mild, non-toxic herb.

COMPLEMENTARY AGENTS: Buchu, Parsley, Uva Ursi, Cranberry, Juniper Berries, Marshmallow, Vitamin C, Bioflavonoids, Proanthocyanidins, B-complex, Vitamin E, Magnesium, Potassium, Copper, Mineral and Electrolyte Supplements

(Also see previous sections on these herbs:GARLIC, QUASSIA, BLACK COHOSH, CASCARA SAGRADA)

THE CARDIOVASCULAR SYSTEM

DISORDERS TARGETED: Heart Disease, Angina, Atherosclerosis, Hypertension, Irregular Heartbeat, Stress, Insomnia, Circulatory Insufficiency

Herbal Formula Five

Hawthorn Berry, Passion Flower, Peppermint, Capsicum, Valerian

Heart Disease is the number one killer of adults in this country. Nearly one million people die annually from cardiovascular-related illness. Our preoccupation with saturated, fatty foods, alcohol, smoking and inactivity has taken an enormous health toll among our population. High cholesterol levels combined with stress and smoking is a most lethal mix and kills thousands of Americans every year. In order to prevent or treat cardiovascular disorders, an effective herbal formula must skillfully combine several herbs, which in tandem, contribute to a healthy strong heart and a competent circulatory system. Cholesterol levels, heart tissue, arterial health and blood pressure must be optimized in order to promote a long and healthy life.

*Hawthorn Berry feeds and strengthens heart muscle and helps to normalize heart rhythms by supporting its metabolic processes.
*Passion Flower promotes relaxation of smooth muscle easing stress and lowering blood pressure.
*Peppermint acts as a catalyst which enhances the action of other herbs.
*Capsicum stimulates and improves circulation, can help decrease blood pressure by lowering cholesterol, and like Peppermint, acts as anl herb activator.
*Valerian counteracts stress calming the central nervous system.

Individual Herbs

HAWTHORN BERRY (CRATEGUS OXYACANTHA)

OVERVIEW: The ancient Greeks were well aware of the Hawthorn Berry and its beneficial effect on the heart. Used in England for centuries to help treat embedded thorns and splinters, Hawthorn Berry was best known for its ability to treat heart ailments. Because it strengthens heart muscle while acting as a mild tranquilizer, it is considered the premier botanical for the treatment of cardiovascular-related disorders.

CHARACTER: cardiac tonic, antispasmodic, astringent, diuretic, sedative

ACTIVE COMPOUNDS: flavonoid glycosides, saponins, procyanidins, trimethylamine, tannins

MEDICINAL APPLICATIONS: angina, irregular heartbeat, blood pressure disorders, congestive heart failure, hypertension, coronary artery disease, high cholesterol, nervous disorders, insomnia, Reynaud's syndrome, sore throat

SCIENTIFIC UPDATES: The cardiotonic properties of Hawthorn are well documented. It is the flavonoid content of Hawthorn Berry that has been clinically shown to dilate peripheral and coronary blood vessels which helps alleviate hypertension and angina.[103] Experimental studies have found that Hawthorn works in three important ways: it eases blood flow, lowers blood pressure and strengthens heart muscle.[104] One of the most desirable benefits of Hawthorn is that its cardioprotective role may actually escalate when used for a prolonged period of time.[105] In addition, Hawthorn has the ability to lower serum cholesterol levels and prevent cholesterol deposits from accumulating in arteries.[106] It is an extremely valuable therapeutic agent for the early stages of congestive heart failure and arrhythmias.[107] Exercise is so important to good cardiovascular health and Hawthorn also helps to more efficiently oxygenate heart muscle under conditions of increased stress.[108]

SAFETY: No known toxicity has been found in Hawthorn. It may potentiate the action of Digitalis and should only be mixed with pharmaceutical drugs when approved by a physician. The effects of Hawthorn can be cumulative.

COMPLEMENTARY AGENTS: Capsicum, Garlic, Passion Flower, Valerian, Peppermint, Gingko, Vitamin C, Vitamin A, Vitamin E, Vitamin B-complex, Calcium/Magnesium, Potassium, Selenium, Coenzyme Q10, Marine Lipids, Phytonutrients

PASSION FLOWER (PASSIFLORA INCARNATA)

OVERVIEW: The blossom of the Passion Flower reminded early Jesuit priests of the crucifixion of Christ, hence the name "passion" evolved. For over two centuries, Passion Flower has been used to tranquilize and naturally sedate agitated nerves. The relaxant properties of Passion Flower are impressive, and like Valerian Root, leave no grogginess or subsequent confusion.

CHARACTER: antispasmodic, nervine, sedative,

ACTIVE COMPOUNDS: glycosides, flavonoids, harmine, harmane alkaloids, maltol

MEDICINAL APPLICATIONS: alcoholism, anxiety, insomnia, nervousness, headaches, hyperactivity, hypertension, cardiovascular disease, asthma, hormonal imbalances, stress

SCIENTIFIC UPDATES: Relatively unknown is the fact that Passion Flower contains low levels of serotonin, a neurotransmitter, which naturally calms the brain, thus achieving relaxation.[109] It is the harmane alkaloids in the herb which have demonstrated their ability to relax smooth muscle and expand the coronary arteries of the heart, thereby decreasing blood pressure.[110] Additional research has also found that Passion Flower exerts an anti-inflammatory action making it useful for conditions like arthritis.[111]

SAFETY: No known toxicity.

COMPLEMENTARY AGENTS: Valerian Root, Hops, Capsicum, Peppermint, Chamomile, Melatonin, GABA, Calcium/Magnesium

PEPPERMINT, CAPSICUM AND VALERIAN (see previous sections on these herbs)

THE RESPIRATORY SYSTEM

DISORDERS TARGETED: allergies, colds, coughs, flu, bronchitis, pneumonia, sinus problems, sore throats, tuberculosis

Herbal Formula Six

Wild Cherry, Capsicum, Mullein, Yerba Santa, Saw Palmetto, Marshmallow, Fenugreek, Slippery Elm, Thyme

In order to adequately treat and protect the respiratory system, a number of functions must be herbally supported. Respiratory disorders are among the most common ailments and are often difficult to cure. An herbal combination designed to therapeutically affect disease needs to not only ameliorate respiratory symptoms, but target the causes of the disease as well. Mucus congestion, allergic reactions, immune system capability and histamine control are targeted by this herbal mix.

Each herb in this formula has been selected for its particular application. Working together, this herbal combination can be quite effective in treating respiratory disorders without the undesirable side effects of conventional drugs.

*Wild Cherry relaxes the nerves which feed the lungs, inhibiting bronchial constriction and cough.
*Capsicum facilitates better circulation, helping to open congested nasal and lung passages.
*Mullein's antispasmodic action helps control coughing and hoarseness; Yerba Santa stimulates the lung to expel mucus.
*Saw Palmetto helps to move out mucus through its diuretic properties.
*Marshmallow's emollient and demulcent attributes soothe sore throats and irritated mucous membranes.
*The high mucilage content of Fenugreek expedites toxins through the colon and helps heal irritated throat and lung tissue.
*Slippery Elm cleanses and eases inflammation.
*The expectorant and antibiotic action of Thyme stimulates the immune system and helps to fight infection.

Individual Herbs

WILD CHERRY (PRUNUS VIRGINIANA)

OVERVIEW: Native Americans traditionally used Wild Cherry Bark to treat lung ailments and diarrhea. Later explorers and colonists became acquainted with its medicinal value and routinely used the bark to create cough elixirs. Extract, poultices and teas made from Wild Cherry Bark have treated all kinds of irritations affecting both the respiratory and intestinal tracts. Today, Wild Cherry is sold in over-the-counter lozenges and cough syrups for its taste component, but is rarely used by conventional medical practitioners in its herbal form. Ironically, it is more esteemed for its flavor than its therapeutic properties. Wild Cherry is usually more effective when combined with other herbs, which boost and augment its actions.
CHARACTER: anti-tussive, aromatic, carminative, expectorant, bitter tonic, parasiticide, sedative stomachic
ACTIVE COMPOUNDS: volatile oils
MEDICINAL APPLICATIONS: allergies, asthma, congestion, coughs, colds, sore throats, bronchitis fever, tuberculosis
SCIENTIFIC UPDATES: Wild Cherry has the ability to calm and soothe irritated mucosal tissue.[112] "Wild Cherry Bark's use for reducing the symptoms of respiratory distress is without equal in the herb kingdom."[113] It can benefit asthmatics by relaxing the nerves which feed the lungs.[114]

SAFETY: No known toxicity.
COMPLEMENTARY AGENTS: Slippery Elm, Capsicum, Fenugreek, Yerba Santa, Mullein, Saw Palmetto, Marshmallow, Thyme, Vitamin C, Bioflavonoids, Proanthocyanidins, Phytonutrients, Vitamin A, B-complex, Vitamin B-12, Potassium, Calcium/Magnesium

YERBA SANTA (ERIODICTYON SPP.)

OVERVIEW: Spanish explorers became acquainted with this plant from American Indians who used the leaves to treat colds, coughs, sore throats, and stomach maladies. Yerba Santa means "sacred herb" in Spanish. One of the primary actions of Yerba Santa is its expectorant effect on upper-respiratory disorders characterized by congestion. Today, the herb is still used in South America to rejuvenate the body in cases of fatigue.
CHARACTER: aromatic, astringent, carminative, expectorant, stimulant, stomachic, alterative
ACTIVE COMPOUNDS: phenolic compounds, free formic acid, volatile oil, phytosterol, resin
MEDICINAL APPLICATIONS: allergies, asthma, bronchial congestion, colds, flu, laryngitis, hemorrhoids, bladder infections
SCIENTIFIC UPDATES: Yerba Santa exerts a strong stimulant action on the lungs enabling them to expel mucus.[115] It also helps to open respiratory passages affected by allergic reactions, and can help decrease nasal discharge.[116] In the past, it has also been recommended for hemorrhoids and bladder infections.[117] In addition, Yerba Santa increases the therapeutic effectiveness of other herbs.
SAFETY: Use in the appropriate dosage.
COMPLEMENTARY AGENTS: Fenugreek, Capsicum, Mullein, Marshmallow, Slippery Elm, Wild Cherry Saw Palmetto, Thyme, Comfrey, Vitamin C, Bioflavonoids, Vitamin A, Calcium/Magnesium, Phytonutrients, Proanthocyanidins

SLIPPERY ELM (ULMUS FULVA)

OVERVIEW: Native Americans used a very healing bark now known as Slippery Elm to treat a variety of skin irritations, wounds and burns. Slippery Elm can promote healing and soothe inflammation due to its high mucilaginous content. Interestingly, George Washington's army ate Slippery Elm bark to sustain life during their winter at Valley Forge. Because it so effectively protects mucous membranes, it has been traditionally used for any kind of tissue inflammation including lung and bowel tissue. Considered one of Mother Nature's best lubricants, Slippery Elm provides excellent therapeutic effects for the respiratory and gastro-intestinal tracts. It is an extraordinary, mild-flavored and highly nutritious herb.

CHARACTER: astringent, demulcent, digestive, emollient, expectorant, mucilant, nutritive tonic, pectoral

ACTIVE COMPOUNDS: mucilage

MEDICINAL APPLICATIONS: abscesses, asthma, bronchitis, colitis, constipation, coughs, diarrhea, digestive disorders, lung ailments, gastritis, ulcers, heartburn,

SCIENTIFIC UPDATES: Clinical studies have proven the value of Slippery Elm for the treatment of diarrhea, coughs, stomach upsets, colitis and a variety of lung problems.[118] The anti-tussive action of Slippery Elm can soothe raw throats and inhibit chronic coughing.[119] In addition, the high mucilage content of this herb helps to heal and restore the mucous membranes of the G.I. tract.[120] The fact that Slippery Elm is found in over-the-counter medications in the U.S. and Great Britain attests to its versatility.[121]

SAFETY: No known toxicity

COMPLEMENTARY AGENTS: Marshmallow, Fenugreek, Saw Palmetto, Mullein, Thyme, Capsicum, Yerba Santa, Wild Cherry, Vitamin C, Bioflavonoids, Vitamin A, B-complex, Vitamin E, Zinc, Acidophilus

THYME (THYMUS VULGARIS)

OVERVIEW: It was the ancient Greeks who named this aromatic plant "thymus" meaning the strength of its invigorating fragrance. Traditionally, it was used as a wound healer and tissue cleanser, however, its ability to act as an antispasmodic in cases of asthma or other lung disorders was eventually discovered. Herbalists consider Thyme as one of nature's most powerful antiseptics. Today, it is commonly used in mouthwashes and topical ointments. Thymol, the main component of Thyme is not only germicidal but can help to expel mucus from the body as well.

CHARACTER: antiseptic, antispasmodic, aromatic, carminative, diaphoretic, disinfectant, expectorant, nervine, parasiticide, sedative, tonic

ACTIVE COMPOUNDS: thymol, saponins, triterpenes, flavonoids, tannins

MEDICINAL APPLICATIONS: bronchitis, coughs, digestive ailments, gas, gingivitis, gout, headaches, laryngitis, lung disorders, sciatica pain, sore throats, stomach problems, throat maladies, worms

SCIENTIFIC UPDATES: The thymol content of Thyme works as an expectorant and cough suppressant and is frequently used in cough syrups prescribed for lung ailments like bronchitis.[122] When combined with Fenugreek, Thyme works to relive the pain of migraine headaches.[123] The carminative properties of Thyme make it an effective treatment for stomach upsets.[124]
SAFETY: Use in appropriate dosages. Check with a physician if pregnant or nursing before taking Thyme
COMPLEMENTARY AGENTS: Fenugreek, Capsicum, Yerba Santa, Marshmallow, Mullein, Saw Palmetto, Wild Cherry, Licorice, Vitamin C, Bioflavonoids, Vitamin A, Acidophilus
CAPSICUM, MULLEIN, SAW PALMETTO, FENUGREEK, AND MARSHMALLOW: (see previous sections on these herbs)

THE RESPIRATORY AND GASTROIN-TESTINAL SYSTEM

DISORDERS TARGETED: allergies, asthma, bronchitis, colitis, colon problems, constipation, coughs, diarrhea, digestive disorders, emphysema, heartburn, infection, intestinal gas, lung ailments, pleurisy, pneumonia, ulcers

Herbal Formula Seven

Pleurisy Root, Blessed Thistle, Catnip, Slippery Elm, Lemon Grass, Sage, Chamomile

Interestingly, herbs that are good for the lungs and related areas are often beneficial to the gastro-intestinal system as well. Because mucous membranes line both the respiratory and G.I. tract, these herbs can perform a dual function. In addition, many health practitioners believe that a malfunctioning colon or an inefficient stomach can predispose the body to lung and sinus infection causing excess mucus buildup and congestion. The following formula addresses both systems and is designed to support, nourish and protect their combined organs.

*Pleurisy Root, an expectorant, works to expel thick mucus from the lungs.
*Blessed Thistle strengthens heart, lung and liver tissue.

*The antispasmodic action of Catnip helps to cleanse the colon and inhibits the formation of gas.
*Slippery Elm, a demulcent, protects and heals inflamed tissue in the lungs and G.I. tract.
*The astringent properties of Lemon Grass inhibit the formation of mucus and help to cleanse the blood of toxins.
*Sage relieves indigestion and inhibits inflammation.
*Chamomile, a nervine herb, calms nerves, eases digestion and reduces fever.

Individual Herbs

PLEURISY ROOT (ASCLEPIAS TUBEROSA)

OVERVIEW: The word "pleurisy" refers to the lungs and indicates the primary therapeutic usage of this herb. Pleurisy Root has been traditionally used to treat pleurisy (an inflammation of the pleural cavity of the lungs), colds, flu, acute bronchitis, chest congestion and pneumonia. Native Americans regarded it as a great healing gift provided by the creator. It's ability to promote sweating has also been valuable in treating the fever which so often accompanies respiratory infections. It also benefits diarrhea, gas and indigestion.
CHARACTER: antispasmodic, carminative, cathartic (mild), diaphoretic, diuretic, emetic, expectorant, nervine, tonic
ACTIVE COMPOUNDS: glucoside (asclepiadin), resins, volatile oil (trace)
MEDICINAL USES: allergies, asthma, bronchitis, emphysema, pneumonia, tuberculosis, cough, sore throat, colds, tuberculosis
SCIENTIFIC UPDATES: Pleurisy Root specifically targets the lungs and stimulates the removal of thick mucus. It helps to mitigate pain and inflammation typical of lung infections. The reputation of Pleurisy Root as an excellent therapeutic for lung ailments extends back for several centuries. Earlier in the century, it was considered the primary expectorant, "acting on organs of respiration, powerfully promoting. . .expectoration."[125] "Pleurisy Root opens up the lung capillaries, which action helps release any thick mucus...thinning it for easier discharge."[126]
SAFETY: Use appropriate dosages as directed
COMPLEMENTARY AGENTS: Sassafras, Slippery Elm, Wild Cherry Bark, Sage, Thyme, Saw Palmetto, Lemon Grass, Blessed Thistle, Mullein, Fenugreek, Capsicum, Marshmallow, Vitamin C, Bioflavonoids, Vitamin A, Calcium/Magnesium, Bee Pollen, Acidophilus

BLESSED THISTLE (CNICUS BENEDICTUS)

OVERVIEW: Ancient Egyptians highly esteemed the seed of the Blessed Thistle plant for its precious oil. In the thirteenth century, physicians of the Myddvai prescribed the botanical for digestive complaints. Over the last several centuries, Blessed Thistle has been used as a tonic for female complaints, headaches and fevers. Its connection with a monastery in Europe during outbreaks of smallpox is thought to have resulted in its "holy" designation.

CHARACTER: alterative, antipyretic, astringent, bitter tonic, diaphoretic, diuretic, emmenagogue, galactagogue, hormonal, nervine, hepato-tonic

ACTIVE COMPOUNDS: sesquiterpene lactone cnicin, lignans, phytosterols, volatile oil, tannins, mucilage

MEDICINAL APPLICATIONS: anorexia, lack of appetite, circulatory disorders, blood purification, cancer, constipation, digestive problems, fever, gallbladder disease, gas, headaches, heart problems, hormonal imbalances, lactation, liver ailments, lung diseases, painful menstruation

SCIENTIFIC UPDATES: Blessed Thistle is an excellent supporting herb for plant combinations. "It helps activate a sluggish liver and corrects stomach and digestive problems, flatulence and tension headaches. It further supports the body's cleansing and detoxifying systems by promoting perspiration and removing excess fluids."[127] Modern studies have found that Blessed Thistle contains antibacterial and anti-yeast properties.[128] It has demonstrated its ability to strengthen the spleen and liver and helps reduce fevers by promoting perspiration.[129]

SAFETY: Ingesting excessive amounts of Blessed Thistle may cause nausea.

COMPLEMENTARY AGENTS: Lemon Grass, Sage, Slippery Elm, Chamomile, Catnip, Peppermint, Milk Thistle, Vitamin C, Bioflavonoids, Calcium/Magnesium, Digestive Enzymes

LEMON GRASS (CYMBOPOGON CITRACUS)

OVERVIEW: Chinese herbalists have used Lemon Grass for colds, headaches, and abdominal cramping. Today, the herb is used to cleanse the blood of impurities. When added to an herbal mix, Lemon Grass works to facilitate the removal of infectious mucus and can help to alleviate stress-related conditions. Its lemony fragrance is due to its citral content, also referred to as Oil of Verbena.

CHARACTER: aromatic, astringent, carminative, expectorant, antipyretic

ACTIVE COMPOUNDS: citral

MEDICINAL APPLICATIONS: colds, digestive upsets, fever
SCIENTIFIC UPDATES: "Lemon Grass is reputed to slow the discharge of mucus, as well as reduce mucus discharge in respiratory conditions, due in part to its astringent properties.[130]
SAFETY: Use in appropriate dosages as directed
COMPLEMENTARY AGENTS: Sage, Blessed Thistle, Marshmallow, Mullein, Pleurisy Root, Catnip, Chamomile, Slippery Elm, Vitamin C, Bioflavonoids, Proanthocyanidins, Vitamin A, Calcium/Magnesium

SAGE (SALVIA OFFICINALIS)

OVERVIEW: For generations, Sage has been associated with longevity and mental acuity. It has been a highly valued herb and in China is used to promote vigor and stamina. In recent times, the energizing properties of Sage have been used as substitutes for caffeine. Sage oil is also utilized in aromatherapy to lift the spirits and invigorate the body. Among its many uses, Sage has the ability to calm a nauseated stomach, soothe a sore throat and treat a cold.
CHARACTER: antipyretic, antiseptic, antispasmodic, aromatic, astringent, carminative, diaphoretic, digestive, parasiticide, stimulant, tonic
ACTIVE COMPOUNDS: diterpene bitters, thujone, cineol, camphor, tannins, resins, flavonoids, saponins
MEDICINAL APPLICATIONS: cankers, coughs, diabetes, digestive disorders, fever, laryngitis, memory, mouth sores, nausea, worms
SCIENTIFIC UPDATES: Sage relaxes peripheral blood vessels, reduces perspiration, salivation and lactation. It is a natural antibiotic and can reduce blood sugar and promote bile flow.[131] The astringent, drying properties of Sage make it useful treating cold symptoms, and relieving the irritation of cankers or mouth sores.[132] Sage is also credited with being a potent antioxidant.[133]
SAFETY: Pregnant or nursing women should check with their physician before taking Sage. Anyone with epilepsy should not use Sage for prolonged periods of time.
COMPLEMENTARY AGENTS: Thyme, Peppermint, Verbena, Ginger, Chamomile, Lemon Grass, Blessed Thistle, Pleurisy Root, Capsicum, Fenugreek Saw Palmetto, Vitamin C, Bioflavonoids, Proanthocyanidins, Vitamin A, Calcium/Magnesium
CATNIP, SLIPPERY ELM AND CHAMOMILE (see previous sections on these herbs)

THE URINARY SYSTEM

DISORDERS TARGETED: bladder infections, kidney disease, incontinence, kidney stones, bed wetting, edema, prostate disorders, water retention

Herbal Formula Eight

Uva Ursi, Parsley, Buchu, Cranberry, Cornsilk, Alfalfa, Marshmallow, Juniper Berry

Urinary system disorders can be linked to a number of factors including poor circulation, inactivity and systemic disease. This particular herbal blend is designed to support and build the urinary system by toning and strengthening the kidney and bladder. Herbs have been selected that can repair damaged tissue, boost blood circulation and increase blood filtration and urine flow.

*Uva Ursi exerts an antiseptic action on inflamed urinary tract mucous membranes and stimulates kidney activity.
*Parsley natural diuretic properties help to cleanse the blood and stimulate the movement of toxins through the kidney.
*Buchu's liptriptic action helps to prevent the formation of kidney stones while it neutralizes excess acidity, thereby reducing the risk of bladder infections.
*Cranberry's antibacterial action fights urinary tract infections.
*Cornsilk heals an inflamed bladder or prostate and inhibits build up of uric acid.
*The chlorophyll of Alfalfa fights infection and cleanses the blood.
*Marshmallow's emollient and demulcent qualities can help ease the passage of kidney stones and soothe inflammation.
*Juniper Berry significantly increase glomeruli filtration in the kidneys, helps to dissolve stones and inhibits water retention.

Individual Herbs

UVA URSI (ARCTOSTAPHYLOS UVA-URSI)

OVERVIEW: Throughout the entire world, Uva Ursi has been used to treat nephritis, kidney stones and chronic cystitis. It's remarkable ability to tone a weakened kidney and stimulate liver and pancreas function make it one of the most valuable herbs in the plant kingdom. Native Americans made Uva Ursi poultices for sprains and sore muscles, however, its real value lies in its ability to cleanse the urinary tract. Marco Polo found that the Chinese called it "the kidney herb." Uva Ursi is an astringent herb with a marked affinity for the organs of the urinary system.

CHARACTER: antilithic, aromatic, astringent, antiseptic, diuretic, urinary tonic

ACTIVE COMPOUNDS: glycosides (arbutin and methylarbutin), quercitin, tannin, hydroquinone, allantoin

MEDICINAL APPLICATIONS: bladder infections, Bright's disease, cystitis, diabetes, nephritis, pyelo-nephritis, water retention, liver ailments, chronic diarrhea

SCIENTIFIC UPDATES: The primary constituent of Uva Ursi is a glycoside called arbutin which is responsible for its diuretic action. In addition, when it is excreted from the kidneys, arbutin produces an antiseptic effect on the mucous membranes of the urinary tract.[134] Chemical compounds in Uva Ursi also help to balance the pH of urine.[135] American research has found that Uva Ursi was effective against nephritis and kidney stones and possessed all-around tonic properties.[136] In addition, tests have found that extracts of Uva Ursi have shown some anti-cancer properties and antibiotic action.[137]

SAFETY: Must be used as directed. Pregnant women should consult their physician before using Uva Ursi. Prolonged or excessive use may cause gastric irritation.

COMPLEMENTARY AGENTS: Parsley, Buchu, Alfalfa, Cornsilk, Juniper Berries, Marshmallow, Cranberry, Lemon Grass, Vitamin C, Bioflavonoids, Vitamin B6, Proanthocyanidins, B-complex, Bee Pollen, Phytonutrients, Mineral and Electrolyte Supplements

PARSLEY (PETROSELINUM SATIVUM)

OVERVIEW: Parsley has a lengthy history of therapeutic use throughout the world. Unfortunately, modern man has relegated it to the status of nothing more than a food garnish. The ancients knew that Parsley could treat kidney and liver ailments and recorded it as a remedy for gallstones. The high chlorophyll content of Parsley gives it an impressive deodorizing action and ability to purify and build the blood. Culpeper wrote that Parsley was an excellent therapeutic herb for all kidney and bladder disorders.

CHARACTER: antiseptic, calcium solvent, carminative, diuretic, nervine, tonic

ACTIVE COMPOUNDS: chlorophyll, flavonoids (apiol, myristicin),

MEDICINAL APPLICATIONS: bed wetting, bladder infections, blood disorders, diabetes, edema, gallstones, halitosis, jaundice, kidney disease, kidney stones, prostate disorders, water retention

SCIENTIFIC UPDATES: Studies have shown that in comparison to citrus juices, Parsley contains three times more vitamin C gram per gram.[138] Recent experiments have established that Parsley can lower blood pressure, kill microbes and tone the uterus.[139] Clinical physicians have also claimed that Parsley is effective as a remedy for liver disease.[140] The flavonoid content of Parsley stimulates urination and provides relief.[141] "Parsley works best in blends with other herbs, such as Buchu and Cornsilk."[142]

SAFETY: Pregnant women should not use excessive amount of Parsley.

COMPLEMENTARY AGENTS: Buchu, Cornsilk, Alfalfa, Uva Ursi, Juniper Berry, Cranberry, Marshmallow, Kelp, Saw Palmetto, Garlic, Vitamin C, Bioflavonoids, Vitamin A, Vitamin E, Zinc, Proanthocyanidins, Bee Pollen, Phytonutrients

BUCHU (BAROSMA BETULINA)

OVERVIEW: Buchu was discovered by the inhabitants of South Africa and has been used as a stimulating tonic and anti-inflammatory agent for the urinary infections. Residents of Cape Colony found that Buchu leaves had a remarkable ability to soothe and heal irritated kidney tissue which had been in contact with highly acidic urine. Today, Buchu is considered one of the most prized and recommended herbs for urinary disorders and prostate disease.

CHARACTER: antiseptic, aromatic, astringent, carminative, diaphoretic, diuretic, urinary antiseptic, tonic

ACTIVE COMPOUNDS: volatile oils, mucilage, diosphenol

MEDICINAL APPLICATIONS: bladder infections, diabetes, kidney disease, prostate disorders

SCIENTIFIC UPDATES: It is the volatile oil content of Buchu which enables it to stimulate urination while acting as a urinary antiseptic.[143] Buchu "acts to eliminate mucus, acid urine and irritation, and is given to combat many forms of inflammation and infection, including cystitis, pyelitis, ureteritis and prosta-

titis."[144] ". . . Diasophenol, which has antiseptic properties is considered by some to be the most important constituent of Buchu."[145]
SAFETY: Use in appropriate doses as directed.
COMPLEMENTARY AGENTS: Uva Ursi, Parsley, Cornsilk, Cranberry, Juniper Berry, Alfalfa, Marshmallow, Bee Pollen, Vitamin C, Bioflavonoids, Proanthocyanidins, Vitamin A, Zinc, Mineral and Electrolyte Supplements

CRANBERRY (VACCINIUM MACROCARPON)

OVERVIEW: Cranberry has been recommended by traditional folk medicine for bleeding gums and other inflammatory conditions. Today pure cranberry juice is prescribed as a preventative agent against the development of bladder infections. The use of concentrated cranberry in capsulized form makes its application more practical and convenient.
CHARACTER: antibacterial, anti-inflammatory, antipyretic
ACTIVE COMPOUNDS: flavonoids
MEDICINAL APPLICATIONS: bladder infections, fever, urinary tract infections,
SCIENTIFIC UPDATES: Recent research suggests that cranberry juice may help fight urinary infections which are caused by certain bacteria.[146]
SAFETY: No known toxicity.
COMPLEMENTARY AGENTS: Parsley, Uva Ursi, Juniper Berry, Marshmallow, Alfalfa, Corn Silk, Vitamin C, Bioflavonoids, Proanthocyanidins, Vitamin A, Zinc, Bee Pollen

ALFALFA (MEDICAGO SATIVA)

OVERVIEW: Alfalfa is frequently categorized as a legume rather than an herb. It has been used for centuries throughout both the Easter and Western world as a remedy for indigestion, and kidney disorders. Arabs referred to Alfalfa as the "father of all herbs" and have cultivated it for hundreds if not thousands of years. After Spanish explorers brought Alfalfa to the New Worlds, it was used to feed livestock. It has not been utilized as a "people food" because humans do not have the capability of breaking down its fiber content. Because it is so rich in nutrients, Alfalfa is considered a panacea for almost every health problem and an effective component of a number of herbal blends.
CHARACTER: alterative, anodyne, anti-acidic, antirheumatic, diuretic, nutritive, stomachic, tonic
MEDICINAL APPLICATIONS: allergies, anemia, arthritis, asthma, Bell's

Palsy, blood disorders, bursitis, cholesterol, diabetes, digestive disorders, fatigue, gout, lactation, kidney disorders, morning sickness, nausea, Cushing's disease, rheumatism, ulcers, urinary tract infections

SCIENTIFIC UPDATES: Alfalfa contains eight essential amino acids, a rich source of Vitamin B-12, natural fluoride and a high chlorophyll content. Alfalfa has demonstrated an anti-rheumatic effect, lowers cholesterol and improves overall health and vigor.[151] Recent French studies have found that Alfalfa can reduce tissue damage caused by radiation exposure.[152] In addition, it has also shown anti-bacterial and anti- tumor properties.[153] Because it can neutralize acidity, it is also beneficial for bladder and urinary tract infections.

SAFETY: Take as directed. No known toxicity.

COMPLEMENTARY AGENTS: Uva Ursi, Juniper, Parsley, Buchu, Cornsilk, Marshmallow, Cranberry, Vitamin C, Bioflavonoids, Proanthocyanidins, Vitamin A, B-complex, Calcium/Magnesium, Marine Lipids, Acidophilus, Phytonutrients

JUNIPER (JUNIPERUS, COMMUNIS)

OVERVIEW: To Native Americans, Juniper tea was a natural remedy for arthritis, colds and stomach pain. The strong, aromatic scent of Juniper was used to ward off the plague in Europe and today, the berry is used for flavoring sauerkraut and gin. Because of its therapeutic properties, Juniper is considered the active plant ingredient in many herbal combinations, included primarily for its diuretic action.

CHARACTER: anti-fungal, antirheumatic, antiseptic (urinary), antispasmodic, aromatic, astringent, carminative, diuretic, stomachic, digestive tonic

ACTIVE COMPOUNDS: volatile oil, glycosides, ascorbic acid, tannin, juniperin, podophyllorixin (anti-tumor constituent)

MEDICINAL APPLICATIONS: adrenal gland disorders, bed wetting, bladder problems, colds, diabetes, fungal infections, hypoglycemia, infections, kidney infections, kidney stones, pancreas deficiencies water retention

SCIENTIFIC UPDATES: Juniper acts directly on kidney function to stimulate urine flow by increasing the rate of glomerulus filtration (blood purification).[154] Studies have found that after kidney disease, Juniper can help restore kidney tissue and normalize blood pressure.[155]

SAFETY: If pregnant, use Juniper only with your physician's permission. Long term or excessive use may cause kidney irritation. NOTE: using Juniper in herbal blends helps to avoid this possibility.

COMPLEMENTARY AGENTS: Cornsilk, Uva Ursi, Cranberry, Parsley,

Alfalfa, Marshmallow, Kelp, Buchu, Queen of the Meadow, Kelp, Vitamin C, Bioflavonoids, Proanthocyanidins, B-Complex, Vitamin E, Magnesium, Potassium, Copper, Mineral and Electrolyte Supplements
MARSHMALLOW (see a previous section)

FEMALE REPRODUCTIVE SYSTEM

DISORDERS TARGETED: hormonal imbalances, infertility, menstrual disorders (PMS, excessive flow, cramps, bloating, fatigue), morning sickness, pregnancy-related problems, menopause (hot flashes, etc.), vaginal infections

Herbal Formula Nine

Dong Quai, Red Raspberry, Damiana, Cramp Bark, Licorice, Sarsaparilla, Queen of the Meadow, Gotu Kola, Squaw Vine, Kelp, Black Cohosh, Saw Palmetto

The primary focus of this herbal combination is to support and strengthen the female reproductive organs and related systems, especially during times of stress. Herbs that target uterine pain, cramping, and muscle tone in combination with herbs designed to correct hormonal imbalances have been selected. Hormonal dysfunction can initiate a whole host of unpleasant symptoms including the miseries of PMS and menopausal transition (bloating, fatigue, depression, mood swings, etc.) In addition to the herbs discussed, plants that naturally energize the body and stimulate the endocrine system have been added to this blend.

*Dong Quai's antispasmodic action helps to relieve menstrual pain while acting as a mild laxative.
*Red Raspberry tonfies and relaxes uterine muscles and helps prevent excessive menstrual flow.
*Damiana exerts a natural anti-depressive action on the nervous system and has been used to treat sexual dysfunction and infertility.
*Cramp Bark naturally relaxes the uterus and is one of the best natural remedies for menstrual pain and heavy bleeding. It also eases the tension and the emotional strain typical in cases of PMS.

*Licorice is considered a uterine and adrenal tonic and helps to stimulate the endocrine system to function more efficiently. It has natural estrogenic properties and helps control blood sugar swings which can occur with PMS.

*Sarsaparilla contains natural progesterone and testosterone agents which helps to adjust hormonal imbalances.

*Queen of the Meadow acts as a natural diuretic helping to alleviate the water retention and bloating associated with PMS and menopausal symptoms.

*Gotu Kola stimulates circulation to prevent varicose veins and energizes the nervous system, helping to treat hormonally induced energy and depression slumps.

*Squaw Vine is considered a uterine tonic which also fights vaginal infections and helps prepare the body for childbirth.

*Kelp assists thyroid function which is intrinsically linked to hormonal health.

*Black Cohosh has the remarkable ability to mimic estrogen in a mild form and can helps remove excess fluid from tissues, while inhibiting menopausal hot flashes.

*Saw Palmetto works very nicely in combination with Dong Quai as a natural anti-inflammatory which helps to correct menstrual dysfunction.

Individual Herbs

DONG QUAI (ANGELICA SINENSIS)

OVERVIEW: Long used in the ancient Eastern world, Dong Quai has a track record as a treatment for menstrual disorders since 500 B.C. Known as Chinese Angelica, it is the most used gynecological herb in China and is prescribed for menstrual cramps, irregular periods and menopausal symptoms. Dong Quai has an impressive reputation for its ability to treat a variety of female complaints including chronic fatigue.

CHARACTER: alterative, analgesic, anti-inflammatory, antispasmodic, blood tonic, diuretic, immuno-stimulant, sedative, uterine tonic

ACTIVE COMPOUNDS: lingustilide, butyl phthalide, butylene, phthalide, ferulic acid, polysaccharides

MEDICINAL APPLICATIONS: atherosclerosis, anemia, bleeding, fatigue, circulatory insufficiencies, high blood pressure, hormonal imbalance, menstrual disorders (irregular periods, painful periods, PMS), menopause, muscle spasms, poor vitality

SCIENTIFIC UPDATES: The chemical constituents of Dong Quai have an immediate stimulatory effect on the uterus by strengthening and normalizing uterine contractions.[156] Both animal and human studies have found the Dong Quai improves peripheral circulation.[157] Research indicates that it is the ferulic acid and lulgustilide content of the herb which prevents spasms and relaxes blood vessels.[158] It also has proven estrogenic activities.[159]

SAFETY: No reported toxicity. Avoid in cases of severe gastro-intestinal disease and check with your physician if pregnant or nursing.

COMPLEMENTARY AGENTS: Kelp, Black Cohosh, Cramp Bark, Squaw Vine, Queen of the Meadow, Sarsaparilla, Licorice, Damiana, Red Raspberry, Licorice, Saw Palmetto, Wild Yam, Vitamin E, Vitamin C, Bioflavonoids, B-complex, Calcium/Magnesium, Potassium, Marine Lipids, Primrose Oil

RED RASPBERRY (RUBUS IDAEUS)

OVERVIEW: Raspberry tea has been a favorite female herbal remedy for generations. Used by Native Americans as an astringent for sore eyes, Red Raspberry can be used as a tonic during pregnancy to strengthen the cervix and tone the uterus. Raspberry vinegars have been used for sore throats and Raspberry leaves for diarrhea and hemorrhoids. Its most popular use, however, has been as a leaf tea taken to prepare for childbirth.

CHARACTER: anti-abortive, analgesic, antispasmodic, astringent, cardiac, diaphoretic, diuretic, laxative, stomachic, tonic,

ACTIVE COMPOUNDS: fragarine (uterine tonic), tannins, polypeptides

MEDICINAL APPLICATIONS: after-birth pains, bowel disorders, childbirth, colds, diarrhea, digestive problems, female complaints, fever, flu, heart disease, lactation, menstrual irregularities, miscarriage, morning sickness, mouth sores, nausea, pregnancy

SCIENTIFIC UPDATES: Research has found that a particular constituent of the Raspberry leaf caused either contraction or relaxation of uterine muscles as needed.[160] "Raspberry leaf temper the effects of hormonal runaway, such as might occur during menstruation, pregnancy and delivery."[161] It is also thought to build the tissue of the cervix to prevent tearing during delivery.[162]

SAFETY: While mild doses are recommended during pregnancy, excessive amounts should be avoided.

COMPLEMENTARY AGENTS: Licorice, Dong Quai, Saw Palmetto, Licorice, Cramp Bark, Damiana, Queen of the Meadow, Squaw Vine, Sarsaparilla, Black Cohosh, Kelp, Gotu Kola, Wild Yam, Vitamin C, Bioflavonoids, B- complex, Folic Acid, Vitamin E, Calcium/Magnesium, Primrose Oil

DAMIANA (TUNERA APHRODISIACA)

OVERVIEW: Traditionally used by the Maya Indians, Damiana was prescribed for lung disorders, vertigo and for its ability to stimulate sexual desire. The British Herbal Phamacoeia lists Damiana as a mild diuretic and laxative. In Germany, official publications have suggested the herb as a treatment for sexual disorders which may lead to infertility. In Mexico, Damiana has been used to treat a number of female problems and to increase sperm count in males. In Germany, Damiana is prescribed for fortification in cases of overwork, or unusual mental stress.
CHARACTER: antiseptic (urinary), aromatic, aphrodisiac, diuretic, hormonal, laxative, nervine, sexual rejuvenator, tonic
ACTIVE COMPOUNDS: volatile oil (betasitosterol), damianin, resins, tannin
MEDICINAL APPLICATIONS: aphrodisiac, bronchitis, depression, emphysema, fatigue, female problems, hormonal imbalances, infertility, impotence, menopause, mood swings, Parkinson disease, PMS, prostate disorders, sexual dysfunction
SCIENTIFIC UPDATES: Clinical studies have found the Damiana benefits sexual debility and nervous tension.[163] Damiana has also been used to treat depression as a "stimulating nervine."[164] It has been applied in cases of chronic fatigue and mental exhaustion.[165] Damiana contains beta-sitosterol ". . . that could have some stimulant effect on the sexual apparatus or could help build sexual health and reproductivity."[166] "It is excellent when used in formulas with herbs such as Ginseng, Suma, Sarsaparilla and Saw Palmetto."[167]
SAFETY: Use in appropriate doses as directed.
COMPLEMENTARY AGENTS: Saw Palmetto, Dong Quai, Red Raspberry, Licorice, Kelp, Sarsaparilla, Black Cohosh, Cramp Bark, Queen of the Meadow, Ginseng, Squaw Vine, Kelp, Gotu Kola, Vitamin E, Bee Pollen, Bee Propolis, B-complex, Calcium/Magnesium, Potassium, Marine Lipids.

CRAMP BARK (VIBURNUM OPULUS)

OVERVIEW: Also known as the Guelder Rose and Black Haw, Cramp Bark has been used since the 14th century when Chaucer recommended its berries. Native American utilized Cramp Bark for conditions where swelling occurred and American Eclectic Practitioners of the 19th century prescribed it for a variety of ailments, particularly to relax the uterus. Regarding Cramp Bark's properties, Finley Elllingwood wrote in 1910, "for sympathetic disturbances of the heart, stomach and nervous system common to ladies." Today, the herb is known as a powerful muscle relaxant.

CHARACTER: astringent, anti-abortive, anti-inflammatory, antispasmodic, diuretic, sedative, muscle relaxant, cardiac tonic

ACTIVE COMPOUNDS: viburnin, valerianic acid, tannins, saponins

MEDICINAL APPLICATIONS: asthma, colic, constipation, digestive disorders, edema, menstrual cramps, muscle cramps, heart disorders, hypertension, leg cramps, nervousness, uterine cramps

SCIENTIFIC UPDATES: Cramp Bark has been referred to as a potent muscle relaxant that has "a very specific action on the uterus and is one of the best remedies for menstrual pain."[168] This herb has been recognized in the National Formulary as a specific antispasmodic also useful for attacks of asthma and hysteria.

SAFETY: Use in appropriate doses as directed.

COMPLEMENTARY AGENTS: Squaw Vine, Dong Quai, Damiana, Red Raspberry, Licorice, Sarsaparilla, Black Cohosh, Peppermint, Vitamin B-Complex, Vitamin E, Vitamin C, Bioflavonoids, Folic Acid, Calcium/Magnesium, Chromium, Selenium, Potassium

LICORICE (GLYCYRRHIZA GLABRA)

OVERVIEW: The history of using Licorice for both medicinal and culinary purposes is lengthy. Even Alexander the Great supplied his soldiers with sticks of Licorice to alleviate their thirst and sustain energy. Glycyrrhizic acid, the primary constituent of Licorice, is 50 times sweeter than sucrose but does not stimulate thirst when consumed. Since 500 B.B., Licorice has been used for stomach ulcers and as a poison detoxifier. It is sometimes called "the grandfather of herbs." Today its use as an adrenal stimulant and uterine tonic is widely known.

CHARACTER: alterative, anti-allergenic, anti-inflammatory, demulcent, emollient, expectorant, hormonal-adrenal, tonic (glandular)

ACTIVE COMPOUNDS: glycyrrhizin, glycyrrhetinic acid, flavonoids, asparagine, iso-flavonoids, chalcones, coumarins, triterpenoid saponins

MEDICINAL APPLICATIONS: Addison's disease, adrenal exhaustion, allergies, arthritis, circulatory insufficiency, colds, coughs, ear infections, fatigue, female complaints, hoarseness, hypoglycemia and hyperglycemia, immune weakness, liver disease, lung problems, ulcers, uterine tonic

SCIENTIFIC UPDATES: Licorice has been the subject of much modern study. It has clearly established its estrogenic activity.[169] The glycyrrhizin content of Licorice stimulates the productions of hormones such as hydrocortisone which work as efficient anti-inflammatory agents.[170] "Studies have shown Licorice to also posses the ability to counter the effects of two tumor producing agents."[171] Licorice has proven anti- inflammatory and anti-allergic properties.[172] The properties of glycyrrhizin contained in Licorice stimulate the production of interferon which boosts immunity.[173] Licorice may also help in the treatment of gastric ulcers and hepatitis.[174]

SAFETY: Licorice should be avoided if high blood pressure is present. Avoid Licorice if you are taking digoxin-based drugs or have rapid heartbeat. Excessive consumption of Licorice can cause symptoms resembling high blood pressure. Taking supplements of Potassium are recommended.

COMPLEMENTARY AGENTS: Wild Yam, Saw Palmetto, Dong Quai, Black Cohosh, Kelp, Gotu Kola, Queen of the Meadow, Sarsaparilla, Cramp Bark, Squaw Vine, Vitamin E, B-complex, Folic Acid, Calcium/Magnesium, Potassium, Phytonutrients

SARSAPARILLA (SMILAX ORNATA)

OVERVIEW: Sarsaparilla grows in regions of Central and South America and has traditionally been used to make root beer, which derives its flavor from the saponins found in the root. It is a valuable herb for achieving glandular balance and also has metabolic-stimulating properties. Sarsaparilla contains natural testosterone and progesterone-like constituents which help to balance out hormonal fluctuations. Today it is used as an overall body and hormonal tonic.

CHARACTER: alterative, antiseptic, aromatic, blood purifier, carminative, diuretic, hormonal, tonic

ACTIVE COMPOUNDS: saponins, parillin

MEDICINAL APPLICATIONS: blood disorders, male and female hormonal imbalances, infertility, menopausal symptoms, joint aches, psoriasis, sexual dysfunction, skin problems

SCIENTIFIC UPDATES: Clinical tests have discovered antibiotic attributes in Sarsaparilla primarily due to its saponin content.[175] Sarsaparilla also has strong diuretic capabilities and dramatically lowers the urea content of the blood.[176] Chinese research has found that as a tonic, Sarsaparilla has value in that it can help rejuvenate the nerves, blood and glands.[177] In Mexico, South America and China, the herb is used to treat infertility.[178]

SAFETY: No known toxicity.

COMPLEMENTARY AGENTS: Saw Palmetto, Licorice, Damiana, Ginseng, Kelp, Squaw Vine, Black Cohosh, Red Raspberry, Bee Pollen, Bee Propolis,

Vitamin E, Vitamin C, Bioflavonoids, Folic Acid, Calcium/Magnesium, Zinc, Marine Lipids

QUEEN OF THE MEADOW (EUPATORIUM PURPUREUM)

OVERVIEW: Also known as Gravel Root, Queen of the Meadow was a favorite therapeutic plant among Native Americans. It was used by a New England Indian healer to treat typhus. As an herbal remedy, Iroquois and Cherokee tribes prescribed it as a diuretic, a burn poultice, and for ailments of the genito-urinary tract. Today, its diuretic action is useful for clearing the urinary tract and for treating prostate disease. It is also used for menstrual pain and to ease childbirth.

CHARACTER: antipyretic, diuretic, expectorant, anti-rheumatic, promotes menstruation

ACTIVE COMPOUNDS: tannins, bitter principle, flavonoids, sesquiterpene lactones

MEDICINAL APPLICATIONS: arthritis, bladder infections, Bright's disease, bursitis, gallstones, gout, joint pain, kidney infections, kidney stones, neuralgia, prostatitis, rheumatism, urinary disorders, water retention

SCIENTIFIC UPDATES: Queen of the Meadow simulates the gland and organs that clear the body of toxic waste.[179] It has been clinically established as a good treatment for rheumatic and gouty joints due to uric acid deposits.[180] It is considered a tonic for the genito-urinary system and can promote suppressed urine flow. [181] Queen of the Meadow works as a therapeutic agent on the uterus and prostate gland.[182]

SAFETY: Take in appropriate doses as directed.

COMPLEMENTARY AGENTS: Kelp, Saw Palmetto, Capsicum, Red Raspberry, Dong Quai, Black Cohosh, Gotu Kola, Damiana, Uva Ursi, Parsley, Vitamin C, Bioflavonoids, B-complex, Vitamin E, Potassium, Magnesium, Copper

GOTU KOLA (HYDROCOTYLE ASIATICA)

OVERVIEW: Considered one of the best herbal tonics, Gotu Kola has been used for centuries to treat nervous disorders, increase mental and physical performance and to rejuvenate and revitalize a fatigued constitution. Today, the herb is prescribed for enhancing the brain, elevating mood and normalizing hormone function. It can help to combat the depression and fatigue that typically accompany PMS and menopause. Gotu Kola is not related to the kola nut and contains no caffeine.

CHARACTER: alterative, antispasmodic, astringent, diuretic, nervine, tonic
ACTIVE COMPOUNDS: asiaticosides, triterpenes
MEDICINAL APPLICATIONS: age related disorders, arteriosclerosis, circulatory problems, high blood pressure, depression, fatigue, hypoglycemia, learning disorders, menopause, nervous conditions, PMS, psoriasis, senility, ulcerations, wounds
SCIENTIFIC UPDATES: Studies have indicated the Gotu Kola works as a tonic for fatigue without the side effects of caffeine.[183] It also stimulates and builds the nervous system counteractingthe effects of stress. Europeans and Asians use this herb for psoriasis, cervicitis and vaginitis.[184] In India, Gotu Kola has enjoyed widespread use as a brain food, with its therapeutic focus on improving memory and promoting longevity.[185]
SAFETY: No known toxicity. Take in appropriate doses.
COMPLEMENTARY AGENTS: Bilberry, Dong Quai, Sarsaparilla, Ginseng, Ginkgo, Capsicum, Licorice, Vitamin C, Bioflavonoids, Vitamin E, Vitamin D, Zinc, Bee Pollen and Bee Propolis

SQUAW VINE (MITCHELLA REPENS)

OVERVIEW: Also called Partridge Berry, Squaw Vine is exclusively associated with Native Americans who used it for any child bearing related purpose. Native American women routinely took Squaw Vine for weeks before their expected delivery dates in order to ensure an easier delivery.
CHARACTER: astringent, diuretic, parturient (childbirth), uterine tonic
ACTIVE COMPOUNDS: saponin, resin, mucilage, dextrin
MEDICINAL APPLICATIONS: childbirth, lactation, menstrual disorders, miscarriage, skin problems, tonic (female), uterine disorders, vaginal yeast infections
SCIENTIFIC UPDATES: Squaw Vine is a natural for herbal combinations designed to correct female complaints or strengthen the female reproductive system. "Squaw Vine is extremely useful for the treatment of water retention."[186] It is accepted as a uterine tonic and a stimulant to the ovaries.[187]
SAFETY: Use as directed in appropriate doses. If pregnant or nursing, check with your physician before using Squaw Vine.
COMPLEMENTARY AGENTS: Kelp, Red Raspberry, Wild Yam, Black Cohosh, Dong Quai, Damiana, Cramp Bark, Licorice, Queen of the Meadow, Saw Palmetto, Vitamin E, Vitamin C, Bioflavonoids, B-complex, Proanthocyanidins, Phytonutrients

KELP (FUCUS VESICULOSUS)

OVERVIEW: Kelp is an excellent source of iodine and is extensively used by the Japanese and Polynesians. It is a plant or herb of the sea and is harvested off the coast of several oceans. In the 1700s, it was used to treat goiter and in 1862, was prescribed for obesity. Kelp is a rich source of vital life-sustaining minerals and nutrients. Because of its high iodine content, it has traditionally been used to treat the thyroid gland, both underactive and overactive types. Kelp also promotes the growth of healthy skin, hair and nails, can rid the body of toxic materials, and has been used to boost mental alertness and uterine disorders. Kelp is an excellent addition to almost any herbal formula.

CHARACTER: alterative, antibiotic, demulcent, diuretic, expectorant, mucilant, nutritive, stimulant

ACTIVE COMPOUNDS: iodine, bromine, alginic acid, alginates

MEDICINAL APPLICATIONS: acne, adrenal insufficiencies, colitis, eczema, endocrine gland disorders, energy, fingernails, uterine disorders

SCIENTIFIC UPDATES: Studies conducted in Japan show a direct correlation between the consumption of algin found in Kelp and the prevention of breast cancer.[188] The ability of algin to stimulate the T-cells of the immune system is thought to be responsible for this effect. The micro-nutrients in Kelp also enhance stamina and help to balance hormones.[189] Tests have suggested that it may also have antibiotic properties.[190] By boosting thyroid function, Kelp may increase energy by regulating metabolism, which may help boost thermogenesis (fat burning).[191]

SAFETY: Use as directed in appropriate doses.

COMPLEMENTARY AGENTS: Alfalfa, Dong Qual, Dandelion, Black Cohosh, Damiana, Gotu Kola, Ginseng, Licorice, Sarsaparilla, Queen of the Meadow, Vitamin A, Vitamin C, Bioflavonoids, Vitamin E, Calcium/Magnesium, Phosphorus, Potassium, Zinc, Phytonutrients, Blue-Green Algae, Bee Pollen

BLACK COHOSH AND SAW PALMETTO (see previous sections on these herbs)

TONIC AND ENERGIZING HERBS FOR ALL SYSTEMS

Herbal Formula Ten

Gimnem Sylvestis, Bilberry, Ginger, Blueberry, Cornsilk, Dandelion, Black Walnut

Stress and fatigue sould be considered modern day plagues which can signif-icantly compromise the quality of our lives. Our battle to feel vigorous enough to tackle the many challenges of daily life must be constantly waged. In addi-tion to a good nutritious diet and adequate sleep, certain herbs can greatly enhance our energy levels and boost our stamina without the side effects of drugs. This herbal blend creates a general energizing tonic for the body.

*Gimnem Silvestis, when used in combination with other herbs, acts to strengthen the entire body by helping to normalize sugar utilization for energy.
*Bilberry's rich flavonoid content strengthens peripheral capillaries allowing for better circulation which enhances cell nourishment.
*Ginger acts as a vascular stimulant and catalyst for other herbs.
*Blueberry's bioflavonoids inhibit inflammation and strengthen the immune system to resist disease and stress related ailments.
*Cornsilk expedites the removal of toxins through the kidneys helping to main-tain pure blood.
*Dandelion is one of the best liver tonics available. Frequently fatigue is due to poor liver function.
*Black Walnut helps to balance sugar levels while it expels toxic materials.

Individual Herbs

GIMNEM SILVESTIS (GYMNEMA SYLVESTRE)

OVERVIEW: This particular herb is primarily used in herbal blend for its tonic action. Its name in Hindu means "sugar destroyer" and is based on its ability to block the action of sugar within the body. It is also thought to inhibit sugar cravings which can lead to weight gain. By blocking some of the absorption of ingested sugar, the risk of dramatic blood sugar fluctuations which can leave the body drained, is lowered when this herb is taken before sugar consumption.

CHARACTER: stomachic, tonic
ACTIVE COMPOUNDS: gymnemic acid
MEDICINAL APPLICATIONS: diabetes, fatigue, hypoglycemia, obesity, sugar cravings
SCIENTIFIC UPDATES: Modern research has found the gymnemic acid, the active ingredient of this herb blocks sugar absorption into the body.[192] A clinical study published in 1986, suggests that extract of Gimnem can significantly enhance liver and pancreatic function.[193]
SAFETY: Diabetics should check with their physician before using this herb.
COMPLEMENTARY AGENTS: Fenugreek, Goldenseal, Milk Thistle, Ginger, Bilberry, Blueberry, Dandelion, Vitamin C, Vitamin A, B-complex, Bioflavonoids, Proanthocyanidins, Chromium, Bee Pollen, Bee Propolis

BILBERRY AND BLUEBERRY (VACCINIUM MYRTILLUS)

OVERVIEW: Because Bilberry and Blueberry are closely related, their attributes will be jointly discussed. Native to Northern Europe and Asia, both berries were traditionally used to treat fragile blood vessels, poor circulation and diarrhea. The components of Bilberry have important urinary antiseptic properties and in World War II were thought to sharpen eyesight and minimize fatigue in British RAF pilots. Today, Bilberry is used to boost circulation, which increases cellular utilization of oxygen and nutrients. It is considered an herbal antioxidant. Blueberry leaves have a long history of folk use in the treatment of diabetes.

CHARACTER: antiseptic, antioxidant, astringent, diuretic, nutritive, tonic
ACTIVE COMPOUNDS: tannins, sugars, fruit acids, glucoquinone, glycosides, myrtillin
MEDICINAL APPLICATIONS: blood sugar, bruising, diabetes, diarrhea, eyesight, gallstones, hemorrhoids, kidney stones, circulatory insufficiency, hypoglycemia, night blindness, urinary disorders, varicose veins
SCIENTIFIC UPDATES: Bilberry is considered an herbal antioxidant which helps to inhibit free radical damage in human tissue. Studies have found that Bilberry extract can kill or inhibit the growth of certain fungi, yeast, and bacteria.[194] Bilberry is also effective in cases of diarrhea and intestinal upset.[195]

Blueberry anthocyanosides have been found to strengthen capillary walls and inhibit free radical damage.[196] In Europe, Blueberry is used to treat diabetic retinopathy.[197]

SAFETY: Diabetics should check with their doctor before taking this herb.

COMPLEMENTARY AGENTS: Goldenseal, Fenugreek, Bilberry, Gimnem Sylvestis, Blueberry, Vitamin C, Bioflavonoids, Proanthocyanidins, Phytonutrients, Vitamin E, A, B-Complex, Chromium, Bee Pollen, Propolis

GINGER (ZINGIBER OFFICINALE)

OVERVIEW: Ginger is one of the most popular culinary and medicinal herbs in the world. Used for thousands of years by both western and eastern cultures, it has treated colds, chills, nausea, and indigestion. Ginger's pungent components are responsible for many of its remarkable therapeutic actions. It is one of nature's most extraordinary botanical medicines. Ginger is frequently added to herbal blends because like Capsicum, it can catalyze and boost the action and potency of the other herbs it combines with.

CHARACTER: analgesic, antacid, anti-emetic, anti-inflammatory, antioxidant, antispasmodic, aromatic, carminative, diuretic, expectorant, stimulant, tonic

ACTIVE COMPOUNDS: phenylalkylketones, (gingerols, shogaols, zingerone), volatile oil (zingiberone, bisavolene, camphene, geranial, linalool, borneol)

MEDICINAL APPLICATIONS: bronchitis, circulation, colds, colic, colitis, diarrhea, fatigue, fever, flu, gas, headache, heart disease, indigestion, morning sickness, motion sickness, nausea, sore throat, stomach maladies, vomiting

SCIENTIFIC UPDATES: Ginger has exhibited some impressive cardio-tonic effects and has also shown its value for alleviating stress and invigorating the body.[198] Numerous scientific studies have been conducted on Ginger. Recent research findings published in Lancet, a medical journal, reported the effectiveness of Ginger in treating motions sickness and nausea over standard drug therapies.[199] Researchers have also found two natural antibiotic agents in Ginger.[200] Ginger as an effective anti- inflammatory has also been confirmed through laboratory tests.[201]

SAFETY: No known toxicity

COMPLEMENTARY AGENTS: Capsicum, Licorice, Peppermint, Garlic, Fennel, Catnip, Bilberry, Dandelion, Black Walnut, Gotu Kola, Kelp, Ginseng, Bee Pollen, Bee Propolis

CORNSILK, DANDELION AND BLACK WALNUT (see previous sections on these herbs)

ENDNOTES

[1] Rebecca Flynn, M.S., and Mark Roest. YOUR GUIDE TO STANDARDIZED HERBAL PRODUCTS. One World Press, Prescott Arizona: 1995.

[2] Ibid.

[3] R. Wohlfart, R. Haensel and H. Schmidt. "The sedative-hypnotic principle of hops (4)." PLANTA MEDICA. 48, 120-123, 1983.

[4] R. Haensel, R. Wohlfart, and H. Coper. "Narcotic action of 2-methyl-3-butene-2-0l contained in hops." ZHURNAL DER NATUERFORSCHUNGEN. 35 c, 1096-1097, 1980.

[5] R. Schaette. DISSERTATION MUENCHEN. 1971, and R. Schaette. "Stable vaerian preparation." GER. OFFEN. 2,230,626, Jan. 10, 1974.

[6] U. Boeters. "Treatment of autonomic dysregulation with valepotriates (Valmane)." MUENCHENER MEDIZINISCHE WOCHENSchrift. 37, 1873-1876, 1969.

[7] V. Kempinskas. "On the action valerian." FAMAKOLOGII I TOKSIKOLOGIIA. 4(3), 305-309, 1964.

[8] R. Klich and B. Gladbach. "Childhood behavior disorders and their treatment." MEDIZINISHCE WELT. 26(25), 1251-1254, 1975.

[9] P.D. Leathwood and F. Chauffard. "Aqueous extract of valerian reduces latency to fall asleep in man." PLANTA MEDICA. 54, 144-48, 1985.

[10] Alma E. Guinness. FAMILY GUIDE TO NATURAL MEDICINE. Reader's Digest Association, New York; 1993.

[11] T. Shipochliev. "Extracts from group of medicinal plants enhancing uterine tonus." VETERINARY SCIENCES (SOFIA). 18(4), 94-98, 1981.

[12] J. Breinlich and K. Scharnagel. "Pharmacological properties of the ene-yne dicloethers from atricaria chamomilla, anti-inflammatory, anti-anaphylactic, spasmolytic, and bacteriostatic activity." ARZNEIMITTEL-FORSCHUNGEN, 18(4), 429-31, 1968.

[13] V. Yakolev and A. Von Schlichtegroll. "Anti-inflammatory activity of alpha-bisabolol, an essential component of chamomile oil." ARZNEIMITTEL-FORSCHUNG. 19(4), 615-16, 1969.

[14] O. Isaac and G. Kristen. "Old and new methods of chamomile therapy. Chamomile as example for modern research of medicinal plants." MEDIZINISCHE WELT. 31(31-31), 1145-49, 1980.

[15] J.L. Hartwell. "Plants used against cancer: a survey." LLOYDIA. 31, 71, 1968.

[16] Guinness, 331.

[17] B.A. Kurnakov. "Pharmacology of skullcap." FARMAKOLOGIIA I TOKSIKOLOGIIA. 20(6), 79-80, 1957.

[18] S. Shibata, M. Harada, and W. Budidarmo. "Constituents of Japanese and Chinese crude drugs. III. Antispasmodic action of flavonoids and anthraquinones." YAKUGAKU ZASSHI. 80, 620-24, 1960.

[19] V. Usow. FARMAKOLOGIIA I TOKIKOLOGIIA. 21(2) 31-34, 1958.

[20] A.F. Gammerman and I.D. Yourkevitch, eds. WILD MEDICINAL PLANTS. Bello-Russia Publishers, Academy of Science, Institute of Experimental Botanics and Microbiology, Minsk: 1965.

[21] T. Usow. FARMAKOLOGIIA I TOXIKOLOGIIA. 21(2), 31-34, 1958.

[22] Ibid.

[23] J.D. Gunn. NEW DOMESTIC PHYSICIAN OF HOME BOOK OF HEALTH. Moore, Wilstach and Keys, Cincinnati: 1861.

[24] James Duke. HANDBOOK OF MEDICINAL HERBS. CRC Press, Boca Raton: 1985, 120.

[25] Michael Murray, N.D., and Joseph Pizzorno, N.D. ENCYCLOPEDIA OF NATURAL MEDICINE. Prima Publishing, Rocklin, California: 1991, 462.

[26] Guinness, 298.

[27] J. Young. AMERICAN JOURNAL OF MEDICAL SCIENCES. 9, 310, 1831.

[28] N. R. Farnsworth and A.B. Seligman. "Hypoglycemic plants." TILE AND TILL. 57(3), 52-56, 1971.

29 P.S. Benoit, H.H.S. Fong, G.H. Svoboda and N.R. Farnsworth. "Biologic and phytochemical evaluation of plants. XIV. Anti-inflammatory evaluation of 163 species of plant." LLOYDIA. 39(2-3), 160-61, 1976.

30 A.R. Hutchens. INDIAN HERBOLOGY OF NORTH AMERICA. Merco, Ontario, Canada: 1973.

31 Edward E. Shook. ADVANCED TREATISE IN HERBOLOGY. CSA Press, Lakemont, Georgia: 1978, 127.

32 Jack Ritchason. THE LITTLE HERB ENCYCLOPEDIA, 3rd ed. Woodland Books, Pleasant Grove, Utah: 1994, 145.

33 P.H. List and L. Hoerhammer. HAGERS HANDBUCH DER PHARMAZEUTISCHEN PRAXIS. Vol. 2-5, Springer-Verlag: Berlin.

34 P. Schauenber and F. Paris. GUIDE DES PLANTES MEDICINALES. Delachaux et Niestle, S.A., Neuchatel, Switzerland: 1969.

35 R.W. Wren. POTTER'S NEW ENCYCLOPEDIA OF BOTANICAL DRUGS AND PREPARATION. 7th ed. Health Science Press, Rustington, England: 1970.

36"Marshmallow" THE LAWRENCE REVIEW OF NATURAL PRODUCTS: FACTS AND COMPARISONS. St. Louis: Dec. 1991.

37 Daniel P, Mowrey. THE SCIENTIFIC VALIDATION OF HERBS. Keats Publishing, New Canaan, Connecticut: 1986, 193.

38 T.V. Zinchenko, and I.M. Fefer. "Investigation of glycosides from betonica officinalis." FARMATSEVT, ZHURNAL. 17(3), 35-38, 1962.

39 Ritchason, 255.

40 "Mullein." THE ST. LAWRENCE REVIEW OF NATURAL PRODUCTS: FACTS AND COMPARISONS, St. Louis: Sept. 1989.

41 James F. Balch M.D. and Phyllis A. Balch, CNC. PRESCRIPTION FOR NUTRITIONAL HEALING. Avery Publishing, Garden City Park, New York: 1990, 56.

42 Mowrey, 76.

43 L. D'amico. "Ricerche sulla presenza di sostanze ad azione anatibiotica nelle piante superiori." FITOTERAPIA. 21(1), 77-79, 1950.

44 F. Ellingwood. AMERICAN MATERIA MEDICA, THERAPEUTICS AND PHARMACOGNOSY. Eclectic Medical Pub. Portland, Oregon: 1983.

45G. Majno. THE HEALING HAND: MAN AND WOUND IN THE ANCIENT WORLD. Harvard University Press, Cambridge: 1975, 217-18.

46 T. Koloata and D. Chungcharcon. "The effect of capsaicin on smooth muscle and blood flow of the stomach and intestine." SIRIRAJ HOSPITAL GAZETTE. 24, 1405-1418, 1972.

47 Paul Barney, M.D. CLINICAL APPLICATIONS OF HERBAL MEDICINE. Woodland Publishing, Pleasant Grove, Utah: 1995, 55.

48 Ibid., 20.

49 Peter Holmes. THE ENERGETICS OF WESTERN HERBS. Artemis Press, Boulder: 1989, 322.

50 Murray and Pizzorno, 419.

51 J. Braeckman. "The extract of Serenoa repens in the treatment of benign prostatic hyperplasia: A multi center open study." CURRENT THERAPY RES. 55, 776-85, 1994.

52 Mowrey, 77.

53 Penelope Ody. THE COMPLETE MEDICINAL HERBAL. Dorling Kindersley, New York: 1993, 79.

54 Murray and Pizzorno, 399.

55 Ody, 79.

56 P,H, List and L Hoerhammer. HANDBUCH DER PAHRMAZEUTISCHEN PRAXIS. Vol. 2-5, Springer-Verlag, Berlin.

57 Mowrey, 75.   58 G.D. Bell and J. Doran. "Gallstone dissolution in man using an essential oil preparation." BRITISH MEDICAL JOURNAL. 278, 24, 1979.

59 Mowrey, 58.

60 M. Marchesi, M. Marcato and C. Silvestrini. "A laxative mixture in the therapy of constipation in

aged patients." GIORNALE DI CLINICA MEDICA. BOLOGNA: 63, 850-63, 1982.

[61] Mowrey, 58.

[62] Murray and Pizzorno, 235.

[63] Flynn, 12.

[64] Ibid.

[65] Ody, 71.

[66] U.C. Bhargava and B.A. Westfall. "Antitumor activity of juglans nigra (black walnut) extractives." JOURNAL OF PHARMACEUTICAL SCIENCES. 57 (10), 1674-1677, 1968.

[67] Mowrey, 230.

[68] Ritchason, 30.

[69] Marchesi, 850-863.

[61] L.O. Lapinina, and T.F. Sisoeva. "Investigation of some plants to determine their sugar-lowering action." FARMATSEVTICCHESKI ZHURNAL. Kiev: 19(4), 52-58, 1964.

[62] Murray and Pizzorno, 419.

[63] Flynn, 12.

[64] Ibid.

[65] Ody, 71.

[66] Bhargava, 1674-1677.

[67] Mowrey, 230.

[68] Ritchason, 30.

[69] S.M. Kupchan and A. Karim. "Tumor inhibitors 114: Aloe emodin: antileukemic principle isolated from Rhamnus fangula L." LLOYDIA, 39, 223-224, 1976.

[70] H.W. Youngken; TEXTBOOK OF PAHRMACOGNOSY. 5th ed. Balkiston, Philadelphia, Pennsylvania: 1943.

[71] P. Behrns. "Healing remedies in word and illustration." KRANKENPFLEGE. 29(3), 101-04, 1975.

[72] Louise Tenney. TODAY'S HERBAL HEALTH, 3rd ed. Woodland Publishers, Pleasant Grove, Utah: 1992.

[73] Ritchason, 66.

[74] Ibid., 68.

[75] M. Grieve, F.R.H.S. A MODERN HERBAL. Dorset Press, New York: 1994, 111.

[76] Barney, 72.

[77] Mowrey, 236.

[78] Ritchason, 190.

[79] Grieve, 663.

[80] Tenney, 114.

[81] Mowrey, 54.

[82] Ritchason, 193.

[83] Mowrey, 54.

[84] Guinness, 308.

[85] Mowrey, 122-123.

[86] C.J. Cavallito and J.H. Bailey. "Allicin, the antibacterial principle of allium sativum. I. Isolation, physical properties and antibacterial action." JOURNAL OF THE AMERICAN CHEMICAL SOCIETY. 66. 1950-51, 1945.

[87] Michael A. Weiner Ph.D. and Janet A, Weiner. HERBS THAT HEAL. Quantum Books, Mill Valley: California: 1994, 160.

[88] Guinness, 308.

[89] Ritchason, 206.

[90] Ibid., 207.

[91] Mowrey, 19.

[92] List, vol. 2-5.

[93] Mowrey, 207.

[94] Ritchason, 260.

[95] L. Kroeber. "Pharmacology of inulin drugs and their therapeutic use. II. Cichorium intybus; taraxacum officinale." PHARMAZIE., 5, 122-127, 1950.

[96] Mowrey, 18.

[97] K. Faber. "The dandelion: Taraxacum officinale Weber." PHARMAZIE. 13(7), 423-435, 1958.

[98] Murray and Pizzorno, 141.

[99] Ritchason, 85.

[100] G. Valette, Y Sauvaire, et al. "Hypocholesterolemic effect of fenugreek seed in dogs." ATHEROSCLEROSIS. 50, 105-111, 1984.

[101] W.A. Thompson. HERBS THAT HEAL. Charles Scribner's Sons, New York: 1976, 160-61.

[102] G. Ribes, Y. Sauvaire, J.C. Valette, et al. "Effects of fenugreek seeds on endocrine pancreatic secretions in dogs." ANNAL OF NUTRITION AND METABOLISM. 28, 37-43, 1984.

[103] Flynn, 47.

[104] Guinness, 311.

[105] "Hawthorn." THE LAWRENCE REVIEW OF NATURAL PRODUCTS: FACTS AND COMPARISONS. St. Louis: May, 1987.

[106] Murray and Pizzorno, 383.

[107] R. Blesken. "Crataegus in cardiology." FORSCHR MED. 110, 290-92, 1992.

[108] J. Kandziora. "The effects of Crataegus on perfusion disorders of the heart." MUENCHEN MEDIZINISCHE WOCHENSCHRIFT. 111(6), 295-98, 1969.

[109] Flynn, 61.

[110] Ibid.

[111] Guinness, 319.

[112] Mowrey, 131.

[113] Ibid. 240.

[114] Barney, 10.

[115] Ritchason, 262.

[116] ibid.

[117] Grieve, 865.

[118] Shook, 163.

[119] Barney, 98.

[120] Ibid., 136.

[121] Ibid., 29.

[122] Guinness, 324.

[123] Velma J. Keith and Monteen Gordon. THE HOW TO HERB BOOK. Mayfield Publishing, Pleasant Grove, Utah: 1984.

[124] Guinness, 324.

[125] Mowrey, 240.

[126] Ritchason, 181.

[127] Barney, 66.

[128] Weiner, 87.

[129] Holmes, 278.

[130] Ritchason, 133.

[131] Ody, 95.

[132] Guinness, 321.

[133] Ritchason, 207.

[134] Ibid., 207.

[135] Ibid., 233.

[136] B.S. Barton. COLLECTIONS FOR AN ESSAY TOWARD A MATERIA MEDICA OF THE UNITED STATES. 3rd ed. Edward Earle and Co., Philadelphia: 1810.

[137] J.L. Harwell. "Plant Remedies for Cancer." CANCER CHEMOTHERAPY REPORTS. July, 19-24, 1960. See also R. Benigni. "The presence of antibiotic substance in the higher plants." FITOERAPIA. 19(3), 1-2, 1948.

[138] Ritchason, 163.

[139] A.Y. Leung. ENCYCLOPEDIA OF COMMON NATURAL INGREDIENTS. New York: 1980, 257- 59.

[140] D.M.R. Culbreth. A MANUAL OF MATERIA MEDIA AND PHARMACOLOGY. Philadelphia: 1927.

[141] Mowrey, 234.

[142] Ibid.

[143] V.E. Tyler, L.R. Brady and J.E. Robbers. PHARMACOGNOSY. 7th ed. Lead and Febiger, Philadelphia: 1976.

[144] H.W. Youngken. TEXTBOOK OF PHARMACOGNOSY. 5th ed. Blakiston, Philadelphia: 1943.

[145] Grieve, 134.

[146] Guinness, 302.

[147] Ritchason, 65.

[148] A.Y. Leung. CHINESE HERBAL REMEDIES. Universe Books, Now York: 1984, 47-49.

[149] Mowrey, 235.

[150] Ibid. 82.

[151] Ibid. 2.

[152] P. De Froment. "Unsaponifiable substance from alfalfa for pharmaceuticals and cosmetic use." FRENCH PATENT 2, 187,328, 1974.

[153] E. Tyihak and B. Szende. "Basic plant proteins with antitumor activity." HUNGARIAN PATENT 798, 1970.

[154] Mowrey, 83.

[155] Ibid., 84.

[156] Flynn, 18.

[157] Ibid.

[158] Ibid., 19.

[159] Murray and Pizzorno, 462.

[160] Mowrey, 186, 109.

[161] Ibid., 109.

[162] Ritchason, 195.

[163] Alma R. Hutchens. INDIAN HERBOLOGY OF NORTH AMERICA. Merco, Ontario, Canada: 1969, 108.

[164] Ody, 164.

[165] Holmes, 300.

[166] L.S.M. Curtin. HEALING HERBS OF THE UPPER RIO GRANDE. Southwest Museum, Los Angeles: 1965.

[167] Tenney, 46.

[168] Ody, 113.

[169] C.H. Costello and E.V. Lynn. "Estrogenic substances from plants: glycyrrhiza glabra." JOURNAL OF THE AMERICAN PHARMACEUTICAL ASSOCIATION. 39, 177-80, 1950.

[170] Ody, 65.

[171] Guinness, 315.

[172] Michael Murray N.D. THE HEALING POWER OF HERBS. Prima Publishing, Rocklin, California: 1992, 160.

[173] "Licorice." THE ST. LAWRENCE REVIEW OF NATURAL PRODUCTS: FACTS AND COMPARISONS. June, 1989.

[174] Guinness, 315.

[175] Mowrey, 19.

[176] Ibid., 19.

[177] Ibid., 287.

[178] Leung, 152.

[179] Mowrey, 4.

[180] Ibid.

[181] J. King. THE AMERICAN DISPENSATORY. Cincinnati: 1866.

[182] Ritchason, 192.

[183] List, vol. 2-5.

[184] ibid.

[185] R.N. Chopra. INDIGENOUS DRUGS OF INDIA. 2nd ed. Arts Press, Calcutta: Chopra R.N. et al. 1933.

[186] Ritchason, 226.

[187] Ibid.

[188] Ibid., 130.

[189] Holmes, 366.

[190] Mowrey, 123.

[191] Ibid., 268.

[192] Betty Kamen. "Gymnema Extract." LET'S LIVE. Sept. 1989, 40-41.

[193] JOURNAL OF ETHMOPHARMACOLOGY. 1986, 143-46.

[194] Weiner, 84.

[195] Rudolf Fritz Weiss. HERBAL MEDICINE. Beaconsfield Publishers LTD., Beaconsfield, England: 1988, 102.

[196] B.O. Bever and G.R. Zahnd. "Plants with oral hypoglycemic action." QUARTERLY JOURNAL OF CRUDE DRUG RES., (17) 139-96, 1979.

[197] IBID.

[198] Mowrey, 104.

[199] Flynn, 28.

[200] "Ginger." THE LAWRENCE REVIEW OF NATURAL PRODUCTS: FACTS AND COMPARISONS: St. Louis: Nov. 1991.

[201] Weiner, 164.